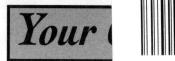

GW00402254

Male & Female
Sterilisation

Jane Smith BSc (Hons)
Medical Editor and Writer, Bristol

&

Alison Bigrigg BM, MRCOG, FRCS, DM, MFFP
Consultant Gynaecologist and
Clinical Director of the Glasgow Centre for
Family Planning and Sexual Health, Glasgow

&

Satyam K. Swami MS, MCh, FRCS Urol.
Clinical Research Fellow, Bristol Urological Institute,
Southmead Hospital, Bristol

ILLUSTRATIONS BY ALEXANDER JAMES

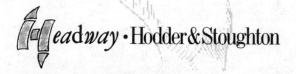

Other titles published in this series

Breast Lumps
Hernias
Hysterectomy & alternative operations
Varicose Veins

Cataloguing in Publication Data is available from the British Library

ISBN 0 340 64374 9

First published 1995
Impression number   10   9   8   7   6   5   4   3   2   1
Year   1999   1998   1997   1996   1995

Typeset by Wearset, Boldon, Tyne & Wear
Printed in Great Britain for Hodder & Stoughton Educational, a division of
Hodder Headline Plc, 338 Euston Road, London NW1 3BH by Cox & Wyman
Limited, Reading.

Contents

General preface to the series   vii

Acknowledgements   x

Preface   xi

Chapter 1   **Introduction**   **1**
The female reproductive organs   1
The male reproductive organs   6
Sterilisation   10

Chapter 2   **Other types of contraception**   **13**
Oral contraceptives   13
Contraceptive injections   14
Contraceptive implants   14
Intra-uterine contraceptive devices (IUCDs)   15
Barrier methods   16
Contraceptive sponges   19
Natural family planning   19

Chapter 3   **Making your decision**   **21**
Discussing sterilisation with your partner   22
When is sterilisation inadvisable?   23
Which partner should be sterilised?   24
Visiting your doctor   26
Physical examinations   27
Visiting the consultant   30
Examination by student doctors   32

	Reversal of sterilisation	32
	Failure of sterilisation	34
Chapter 4	**Going in to hospital**	**36**
	Day-case surgery	37
	Hospital staff	38
	Operations involving a general anaesthetic	41
	Smoking	48
	Obesity	48
	Waiting	48
	Leaving the ward for your operation	49
Chapter 5	**Anaesthesia**	**50**
	Local anaesthesia	50
	General anaesthesia	51
	Pain relief	56
Chapter 6	**The operation: vasectomy**	**58**
Chapter 7	**The operation: tubal ligation**	**61**
	Laparoscopic sterilisation	62
	Laparotomy	68
Chapter 8	**After your operation**	**72**
	After vasectomy	72
	After tubal ligation	74
Chapter 9	**Possible complications**	**78**
	General complications	78
	Following vasectomy	79
	Following tubal ligation	82
Chapter 10	**Private care**	**85**
	Private health insurance	85

Fixed Price Care   86
Arranging the operation   88
Admission to hospital   89
Preparing for your operation   90
Discharge from hospital   90
Differences and similarities   90
Summary   91

Appendix I **Questions and answers**   **93**

Appendix II **Case histories**   **101**

Appendix III **Medical terms**   **109**

Appendix IV **How to complain**   **122**
Hospital staff   123
The Hospital General Manager   123
District Health Authority   124
Community Health Council   125
Regional Medical Officer   125
Family Health Services Authority   125
Health Service Commissioner   125
Taking legal action   127
Summary   127

Index   129

General preface to the series

Two people having the same operation can have quite different experiences, but a feeling that is common to many is that things might have been easier if they had had a better idea of what to expect. Some people are reluctant to ask questions, and many forget what they are told, sometimes because they are anxious, and sometimes because they do not really understand the explanations they are given.

The emphasis in most medical centres in Britain today is more on patient involvement than at any time in the past. It is now generally accepted that it is important for people to understand what their treatment entails, both in terms of reducing their stress and thus aiding their recovery, and of making their care more straightforward for the medical staff involved.

The books in this series have been written with the aim of giving people comprehensive information about each of the medical conditions covered, about the treatment they are likely to be offered, and about what may happen during their post-operative recovery period. Armed with this knowledge, you should have the confidence to question, and to take part in the decisions made.

Going in to hospital for the first time can be a daunting experience, and therefore the books describe the procedures involved, and identify and explain the roles of the hospital staff with whom you are likely to come into contact.

Anaesthesia is explained in general terms, and the options

available for a particular operation are described in each book.

There may be complications following any operation – usually minor but none the less worrying for the person involved – and the common ones are described and explained. Now that less time is spent in hospital following most non-emergency operations, knowing what to expect in the days following surgery, and what to do if a complication does arise, is more important than ever before.

Where relevant, the books include a section of exercises and advice to help you to get back to normal and to deal with the everyday activities which can be difficult or painful in the first few days after an operation.

Doctors and nurses, like members of any profession, use a jargon, and they often forget that many of the terms that are familiar to them are not part of everyday language for most of us. Care has been taken to make the books easily understandable by everyone, and each book has a list of simple explanations of the medical terms you may come across.

Most doctors and nurses are more than willing to explain and to discuss problems with patients, but they often assume that if you do not ask questions, you either do not want to know or you know already. Questions and answers are given in every book to help you to draw up your own list to take with you when you see your GP or consultant.

Each book also has a section of case histories of people who have actually experienced the particular operation themselves. These are included to give you an idea of the problems which can arise, problems which may sometimes seem relatively trivial to others but which can be distressing to those directly concerned.

Although the majority of people are satisfied with the medical care they receive, things can go wrong. If you do feel you need to make a complaint about something that happened, or did not happen, during your treatment, each book has a section which deals in detail with how to go about this.

It was the intention in writing these books to help to take some of the worry out of having an operation. It is not knowing what to expect, and the feeling of being involved in some process over which we have no control, and which we do not fully understand, that makes us anxious. The books in the series *Your Operation* should help to remove some of that anxiety and make you feel less like a car being serviced, and more like part of the team of people who are working together to cure your medical problem and put you back on the road to health.

You may not know *all* there is to know about a particular condition when you have read the book related to it, but you will know more than enough to prepare yourself for your operation. You may decide you do not want to go ahead with surgery. Although this is not the authors' intention, they will be happy that you have been given enough information to feel confident to make your own decision, and to take an active part in your own care. After all, it is *your* operation.

Jane Smith
Bristol, 1995

Acknowledgements

We are grateful to various people for their help and advice during the writing of this book. We would particularly like to thank Mr David J. Leaper, FRCS, Consultant and Senior Lecturer in Surgery at Southmead Hospital and the University of Bristol; Dr Alasdair Dow, FRCA, Consultant in Anaesthesia and Intensive Care at the Royal Devon and Exeter Hospital; and Ward Sisters Dorothy Lockett and Carol Blunsum at Southmead Hospital, Bristol.

Thanks are also due to the men and women whose experiences we have related in the section of case histories.

Preface

When the contraceptive pill first became widely available to women, it was seen by many as the definitive answer to the problem of contraception. However, within a few years, some potentially harmful effects of the high doses of hormones used in the early pills began to become apparent. Although many of the problems have now been overcome with the much lower doses of hormones in modern-day pills, their long-term use is still not advisable for some women, and many others do not wish to take them. Consequently, sterilisation has become an increasingly popular alternative in recent years, although the newer contraceptive methods involving implants and injections are also beginning to be used more widely.

The sterilisation operation for men is a quick and simple procedure which is normally done using a local anaesthetic. For women, a general anaesthetic is usually required, but the relatively recent introduction of the use of laparoscopic surgery for female sterilisation means that, where this is available, the post-operative recovery time has been reduced for women too.

However, there are important factors to be considered by anyone contemplating sterilisation, and the operation and its implications should be clearly understood – by both partners in a relationship – before this decision is made. Your GP or a doctor at a family planning clinic should be able to offer you advice and information, but the final decision is yours, ideally made together with your partner.

Although reversal of a sterilisation operation is theoretically possible, the surgery it involves is complicated and often unsuccessful, and it is thus necessary for this method of contraception to be viewed as irreversible.

We hope that this book will provide you with enough information about all aspects of male and female sterilisation to be confident of making an informed decision which is right for you.

Jane Smith
Alison Bigrigg
Satyam K. Swami
1995

CHAPTER 1

Introduction

Sterilisation differs from other types of contraception in that it involves a surgical procedure and must always be considered to be irreversible.

Before looking at what is involved in the sterilisation operations for men and women, and in making the decision to opt for this form of contraception, it is helpful to have some understanding of the structure and function of the male and female reproductive organs.

THE FEMALE REPRODUCTIVE ORGANS

The ovaries

Each of the two ovaries is a solid, almond-shaped organ which, after puberty, is about 3.5 cm (1.5 inches) long. The ovaries are attached to the side walls of the pelvic cavity by ligaments, and each is situated near the open end of a fallopian tube (see below).

When a female child is born, her ovaries already contain several thousand microscopic **ova**, the female eggs. Each ovum is surrounded by a blister-like **ovarian follicle**. Although the ova themselves do not increase in size, some of the follicles mature and enlarge at puberty, surrounding the ova within them with fluid.

Throughout a woman's reproductive life, from puberty to the menopause, **ovulation** occurs in the middle of each menstrual cycle when a mature follicle ruptures within an ovary, releasing its ovum. The ovum then normally passes into the adjacent fallopian tube and begins its journey towards the uterus. The remains of the ruptured ovarian follicle form a yellow body, the **corpus luteum**, which produces the hormone **progesterone**, the action of which helps to prepare the lining of the womb for pregnancy.

The fallopian tubes

Each of the two fallopian tubes is about 10 cm (4 inches) long, and has tiny hair-like structures around its opening which help to waft the released ovum into it. Fertilisation of an ovum by a sperm normally occurs within a fallopian tube, and the fertilised egg then continues along the tube to the uterus.

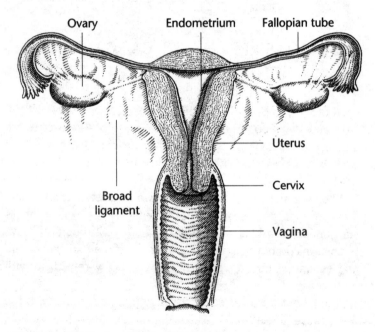

The internal female reproductive organs.

The uterus

The uterus, or womb, is a pear-shaped organ, about 7.5 cm (3 inches) long after puberty. It has thick muscular walls, the **myometrium**, surrounding a cavity. The uterine cavity is lined by blood-rich tissue called the **endometrium**, the surface layer of

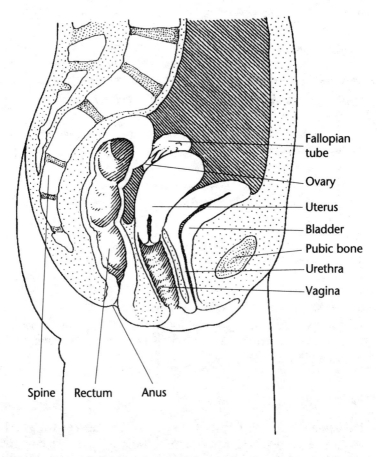

Fallopian tube

Ovary

Uterus

Bladder

Pubic bone

Urethra

Vagina

Spine   Rectum   Anus

The position of the female internal reproductive organs in relation to the bladder and rectum.

3

which is shed during each menstrual period. If a fertilised ovum becomes implanted in the endometrium, the menstrual periods cease and, instead of being shed, the endometrium remains to provide a suitable surface for the development of the fetus.

The uterus forms a protected environment for a developing fetus, and can increase in size by some thirty times during pregnancy. Its muscular walls contract during labour to push the baby down the birth canal.

After puberty, the uterus mainly consists of the body, or **corpus**, the remainder forming the neck, or **cervix**, which protrudes into the top of the vagina. The part of the uterus above its two upper corners into which the fallopian tubes open is known as the **fundus**.

Secretions from glands within the cervical canal help to keep the vagina sterile. The cervical mucus, which normally forms a barrier against sperm, becomes thinner during the fertile phase of the menstrual cycle, thus allowing sperm to penetrate through the cervix into the body of the uterus and reach the fallopian tubes.

The vagina

The vagina is a sensitive, muscular canal which extends from the uterus to an external opening, the **introitus**, in the **vulva**. It is approximately 10 cm (4 inches) long, although its length varies from woman to woman. The vagina is kept moist by secretions from glands within the cervix.

Menstruation

Menstruation usually begins in girls in the UK between the ages of 10 and 16. Each menstrual cycle starts on the first day of menstrual bleeding, and ends on the day before the next period of bleeding begins. The length of the menstrual cycle varies from

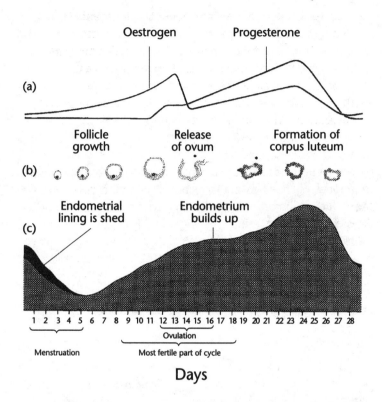

(a)

Oestrogen   Progesterone

Follicle
growth

Release
of ovum

Formation of
corpus luteum

(b)

Endometrial
lining is shed

Endometrium
builds up

(c)

1 2 3 4 5 6 7 8 9 10 11 12 13 14 15 16 17 18 19 20 21 22 23 24 25 26 27 28

Ovulation

Menstruation   Most fertile part of cycle

Days

The menstrual cycle. This diagram shows what happens during a typical menstrual cycle of 28 days. The length of the cycle will vary from woman to woman. (a) Fluctuation in the levels of the hormones oestrogen and progesterone throughout a complete menstrual cycle. (b) A follicle enlarges in the ovary and, at ovulation, ruptures to release its ovum. The remains of the follicle then form the corpus luteum. (c) The outer layer of endometrium is shed during menstruation, after which the endometrial lining of the womb builds up again as it prepares for the possible implantation of a fertilised egg. If no egg implants, the cycle starts again, with the shedding of the endometrium.

woman to woman, the average being about 28 days. It is controlled by hormones produced in the pituitary gland in the brain – follicle-stimulating hormone (FSH) and luteinising hormone (LH) – and it is the action of these hormones which controls the development of ovarian follicles and the maturation and release of the ova. If an ovum fails to become fertilised and to implant in the endometrium after its release from the ovary, menstrual bleeding occurs 14 days after ovulation as the endometrium is shed.

The menopause marks the end of a woman's reproductive life: hormonal changes take place, menstruation ceases, and the reproductive organs gradually start to shrink. For women in Western Europe, the menopause normally occurs between the ages of 49 and 51.

THE MALE REPRODUCTIVE ORGANS

The prostate

The prostate is a glandular organ, about the size and shape of a chestnut, which is enclosed in a fibrous capsule and surrounds the base of the bladder. Enlargement of the prostate gland is common in men as they get older and, because of its proximity to the urethra, this can lead to problems with the passage of urine.

The male urethra

In both men and women, urine is discharged from the bladder via the urethra. In men, the urethra has the additional function of transporting semen. The male urethra is a canal about 20 cm (8 inches) long which extends from the neck of the bladder to the bulbous tip of the penis.

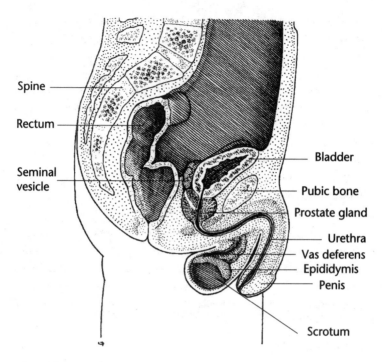

Spine

Rectum

Seminal
vesicle

Bladder

Pubic bone

Prostate gland

Urethra

Vas deferens

Epididymis

Penis

Scrotum

The male reproductive organs.

Testes

Each of the two testes is an oval, glandular organ about 4 cm
(1.5 inches) long by 2.5 cm (1 inch) wide. The testes develop in a
fetus near the kidneys, but by birth each has normally
descended through the **inguinal canal** in the abdominal wall
and into the **scrotum**. As each testis descends, it draws
down with it its blood, nerve and lymphatic supplies, which
together form the **spermatic cord**. The two testes are separated
within the scrotum, and each is contained within a fibrous
capsule.

7

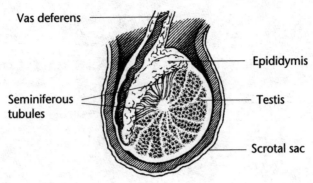

The scrotal sac.

Each testis is divided into approximately 200 to 300 lobules, and each lobule contains one to three tightly coiled **seminiferous tubules**, in which sperm are produced. The seminiferous tubules are the first in a system of ducts through which sperm are transported from the testes to the urethra in the penis.

Epididymis

There is an epididymis alongside each testis which consists of a coiled tube, about 6 m (6.5 yards) long when extended. Sperm pass from the seminiferous tubules within the testis to the coiled **efferent duct** which forms the head region of each epididymis. Apart from the enlarged head region, the epididymis has a body and a tapering tail region.

Vas deferens

The efferent duct emerges from the tail of each epididymis to form a vas deferens, a cord-like duct about 45 cm (18 inches) long. Each vas deferens (plural: vasa deferentia) passes along the scrotum to join a spermatic cord, and thence a **seminal vesicle**. Each of the two seminal vesicles, which lie at the base

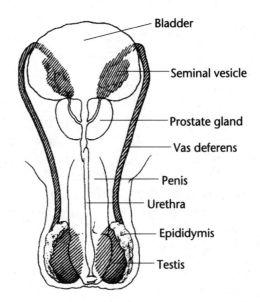

Bladder

Seminal vesicle

Prostate gland

Vas deferens

Penis

Urethra

Epididymis

Testis

The male genital tract. This is a schematic representation; the bladder as shown here is empty and will expand when full of urine.

of the bladder adjacent to the prostate gland, is a coiled tube, about 5 cm (2 inches) long, which acts as a store for semen. Semen enters the urethra via an **ejaculatory duct**.

The penis

The penis is composed of three cylinders of erectile tissue enclosed within a tubular sheath. When ejaculation occurs following sexual arousal, semen is discharged via the ejaculatory duct into the upper part of the urethra and is ejected through the lower, penile part. Semen is prevented from passing into the bladder during ejaculation by the contraction of a ring of muscle around its base.

Sperm

Sperm produced in the seminiferous tubules mature in the epididymis. The production of sperm is continuous, and it takes about three months for them to mature and develop. They then pass through the network of tubes described above, to be stored in the seminal vesicles near the prostate gland. When a man has an erection during sexual activity, large numbers of sperm leave the seminal vesicles and, together with secretions from the prostate, enter the urethra as semen. When ejaculation occurs, the contractions of the muscles around the penis cause the semen to be expelled.

Sperm which are ejaculated into a woman's vagina pass through the cervix into her womb, and thence to the fallopian tubes.

STERILISATION

Any decision to undergo a sterilisation operation should be considered carefully, preferably by both partners in a relationship, and the various factors which need to be taken into account are dealt with in Chapter 3. More detailed explanations of the operations outlined briefly below can be found in Chapters 6 and 7.

Female sterilisation

Fertilisation of an ovum by a sperm normally occurs within one of the fallopian tubes, the passageways of which are no wider than a hair. The sterilisation operation for a woman therefore involves closing both fallopian tubes, usually by placing a clip or ring across each one (**tubal ligation** or **occlusion**) or removing part of them (**segmental excision**). Ligation of the fallopian tubes has the effect of occluding them, and although the former term is used in this book, the two are often used inter-changeably. Tubal ligation is normally done using an instrument called a laparoscope (see p.62), whereas segmental excision involves the more invasive operation known as laparotomy (see p.68).

Following either type of operation, ovulation will continue each month, although the tiny ova released into the fallopian tubes from the ovaries will no longer be able to continue their passage along the tube, and will simply be absorbed by the body.

Sterilisation does not have any affect on a woman's periods. If you have very heavy periods and wish to be sterilised, **hysterectomy** may be more appropriate, and you should discuss this possibility with your GP. However, hysterectomy is a major operation, involving the removal of the womb itself, and it would not be considered as a means of sterilising a woman unless she had other menstrual problems.

Tubal ligation can often be done as day-case surgery (see p.37), and otherwise rarely involves more than one night in hospital post-operatively. You will, however, have to remain in hospital until you have fully recovered from the immediate effects of the general anaesthetic used. Being a more invasive procedure, laparotomy for segmental excision involves a stay in hospital of two to three days.

Male sterilisation

Male sterilisation is known as **vasectomy**. It involves the surgical removal of a small portion of each vas deferens between the testis and the urethra. Like female sterilisation, the operation has to be bilateral, i.e. performed on the vasa deferentia from both the left and right testes.

As vasectomies are normally done under local anaesthetic, they can be performed in out-patient clinics or sometimes in

GP surgeries or family planning clinics which have a small operating theatre. You can usually go home within an hour or two after your operation.

Sperm continue to be produced in the seminiferous tubules following vasectomy, but are absorbed by the body.

CHAPTER 2

Other types of contraception

There are various contraception methods available, and family planning services are provided free under the NHS – mainly by GPs, family planning clinics or voluntary organisations such as the Brook Advisory Centres.

You should consider the alternatives before you start to think about sterilisation, and this chapter provides brief details of different types of contraception.

ORAL CONTRACEPTIVES

Oral contraceptives may be combined – containing synthetic derivatives of the hormones oestrogen and progesterone (the latter known as progestogen) – or progestogen-only pills. Modern oral contraceptives contain much lower doses of hormones than did the early types, and are considered to be much safer.

The combined forms constitute one of the most effective reversible methods of contraception, but the pills do have to be taken regularly each day.

The synthetic hormones contained in these contraceptive pills prevent ovulation, stop changes occurring in the endometrium which are necessary for implantation of a fertilised ovum, and alter the cervical mucus to inhibit penetration by sperm.

Minor side-effects such as headaches, fluid retention and weight gain can develop in women taking oral contraceptives, but more serious complications are uncommon. However, some women with certain risk factors such as existing heart disease or previous thrombosis should not take oral contraceptives.

The progestogen-only pills are useful for women who cannot be given oestrogen, for example those over 35 who are heavy smokers or those who are breast-feeding. They are, however, less effective than the combined pills.

CONTRACEPTIVE INJECTIONS

There are two contraceptives currently available in the UK for intramuscular injection – Depo-Provera and Noristerat. The effects of the former last for 12 weeks, the latter for eight. They are very effective and overcome the need to have to remember to take a daily oral pill.

The injections seem to have only minor side-effects, mostly similar to those associated with the oral contraceptives, but they may cause irregular menstrual bleeding in some women. When the contraceptive injections are stopped, there can be a delay of up to a year or more before fertility returns. As with the oral contraceptives, some women are unsuited to this method, for example those with previous severe arterial disease.

CONTRACEPTIVE IMPLANTS

Norplant is the most commonly used of the contraceptive hormone implants in the UK. It consists of thin flexible rods, each about 3.5 mm long by 2.5 mm wide, containing the hormone levonorgestrel.

Norplant is inserted through a small incision made in the arm above the elbow under local anaesthetic, and remains effective for five years, slowly releasing its content of hormone. It acts by preventing ovulation in some menstrual cycles, and by thickening the cervical mucus to block the passage of sperm into the womb.

Contraceptive implants are very effective, their possible side-effects being minor and similar to those of the progestogen-only pill. They may, however, cause irregular menstrual bleeding in some women. Fertility returns once the implant is removed.

INTRA-UTERINE CONTRACEPTIVE DEVICES (IUCDS)

An IUCD, or coil, is a plastic device which must be inserted into a woman's uterus by a specially trained doctor. Coils tradition-ally contain copper which is slowly released to prevent implan-tation of a fertilised egg in the womb. A new type of coil will soon be available which releases the synthetic hormone progestogen instead of copper and which will not only act as a contraceptive, but will also be useful for women with menstrual problems as it reduces the amount of menstrual blood loss.

Coils have small threads attached to them which come through the cervix and can be felt by the woman to check that the device remains in place.

For young women, IUCDs need to be replaced every five years. Those inserted after the age of 40 may be left until the menopause.

Coils can cause irregular or heavy periods, particularly for the first couple of months after insertion, and may have a small associated risk of causing pelvic infection. Particularly when used by women who have not had children, the devices may be spontaneously expelled.

If pregnancy does occur when an IUCD is in place, complica-tions can arise, sometimes with the fertilised egg developing in a fallopian tube rather than in the uterus – an **ectopic preg-nancy**. Ectopic pregnancies can also occur following female sterilisation operations.

BARRIER METHODS

Diaphragms and caps

There are various different types of caps and diaphragms which can be inserted into the vagina to fit over the cervix and thus prevent sperm passing into the uterus and reaching an ovum. They should always be used with a spermicide (see p.18), be inserted before sexual intercourse, and be left in place for at least six hours after intercourse, and for no more than 30.

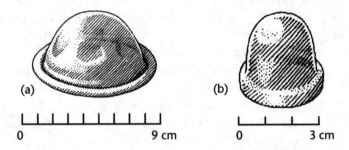

(a)   (b)

0   9 cm   0   3 cm

(a) **A diaphragm.** Diaphragms are available in a range of sizes, from 6 to 9 cm across. (b) **A cervical cap.** Caps vary in size from 2 to 3 cm across.

Once your first diaphragm or cervical cap has been fitted and the right size selected for you, you will be taught how to insert and remove it yourself, and how to check it before intercourse to make sure that it has not become accidentally dislodged.

Diaphragms and caps are effective means of contraception when used correctly, and have few side-effects. However, some women may be allergic to the device itself or to the spermicide. Infection of the urinary tract such as cystitis can occur, possibly due to the pressure caused by a diaphragm or cap which is too big.

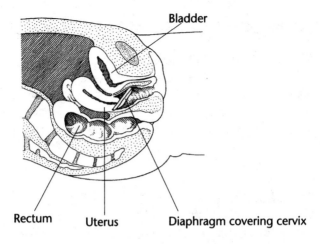

A diaphragm in position. One end of the diaphragm covers the cervix, and the other rests against the pubic bone, thus blocking the entry of sperm into the uterus.

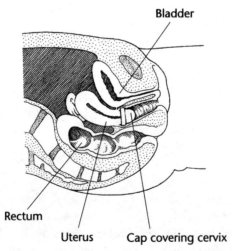

A cervical cap in position. The cap covers the cervix, thus providing a physical barrier to entry of sperm into the uterus.

17

Female condoms

A polyurethane sheath attached to two flexible rings can be inserted into the vagina before intercourse to line it and prevent sperm entering the uterus. This method has no known side-effects, and is quite effective if used correctly. The female condom – available in the UK as Femidom – can only be used once.

Male condoms

Apart from vasectomy, the male condom is the only reliable contraceptive which can be used by a man. The condom is a latex sheath which is fitted over the penis when erect, and which collects ejaculated semen, thereby preventing it entering the woman's vagina.

With correct and careful use, this is an effective contraceptive method, with no side-effects other than occasionally causing irritation or an allergic reaction to the sheath itself or to the spermicide if used.

Apart from acting as a contraceptive, the condom is a means of preventing the transference of the HIV (AIDS) virus and other infections between sexual partners.

Spermicides

Spermicides are chemicals in the form of foams, jellies, creams etc. which are inserted into the vagina before intercourse and which kill sperm. They should be used with one of the barrier methods of contraception described above. Some people dislike using spermicides as they consider them to be messy. In some cases they can cause sensitivity or irritation.

CONTRACEPTIVE SPONGES

A small, round, foam sponge, impregnated with spermicide, can be inserted into the vagina before sexual intercourse. The sponge has a thread attached to aid its removal. Once moistened, the spermicide becomes active, and the sponge itself can also absorb some of the semen which enters the vagina. The sponge also acts as a physical barrier by covering the cervix.

Contraceptive sponges are not very effective, but may be suitable for women whose fertility is reduced, for example those who are breast-feeding or approaching their menopause.

The sponge must remain in place for at least six hours after intercourse, and should not be used during a menstrual period.

NATURAL FAMILY PLANNING

The natural methods of family planning depend on a woman being able to recognise the signs of ovulation, knowing when the different phases of her menstrual cycle will occur, and avoiding having sexual intercourse during her fertile phase. They include the following.

* *The temperature method*. Body temperature varies slightly at different stages of the menstrual cycle, and this method involves the woman understanding and detecting the temperature changes which occur after ovulation.
* *The cervical mucus method*. This involves the woman detecting changes in the consistency of cervical mucus which occur at different phases of the menstrual cycle.
* *The calendar method*. Noting the dates of the different phases of your menstrual cycle over several months can allow you to calculate the probable time of your fertile phase. However, this method is now considered to be unreliable as it does not take into account the various factors which can affect the menstrual cycle such as stress or illness.

* *The double-check method.* A combination of the other three methods, this relies on women observing their own bodies and keeping menstrual records to chart their fertile and infertile phases. It is thought to be the most effective of the natural family planning methods if learned from a specially trained teacher.

The above are only summaries of different contraceptive methods, and your GP or a doctor at a family planning clinic will be able to give you more detailed explanations if you wish to know more about any of them.

CHAPTER 3

Making your decision

Before being able to make a fully informed decision about whether sterilisation is an appropriate form of contraception for you, there are various factors which need to be taken into account.

It is important that, if at all possible, the decision to be sterilised should be a joint one, made by both the partners in a couple. Although it is no longer necessary to obtain your partner's signed consent before you can be sterilised, it is quite common for marriages to suffer, and even to break down, if men or women go ahead with the operation against their partners' wishes. It is also better for both partners to talk things through with their doctor, taking account of the advice they may be offered.

Before choosing sterilisation as a means of contraception, all other methods of family planning should be considered, and perhaps discussed with your GP or a doctor at a family planning clinic (see Chapter 2).

Once you have decided you want to be sterilised, you should make an appointment to talk to your GP or a doctor at a family planning clinic – preferably together with your partner – who will probably refer you to a consultant surgeon at a hospital or health centre where the operation can be performed. However, a vasectomy can often be carried out without the need for prior discussion with a consultant. Exceptions to this are men who have had previous scrotal surgery, infection of the epididymis (**epididymitis**) or a hernia repair operation. They will probably need to be examined by a consultant, or a doctor on the consultant's team, before they attend for their operation. Any scar tissue resulting from a previous operation or infection may make operating under local anaesthetic more difficult, and a general anaesthetic may have to be used instead.

Although it is not always the case, you are likely to be questioned carefully by your GP, and again by the consultant if you see one. The decision as to which partner is sterilised is a matter of individual choice, and some people may find such questioning embarrassing, or even intrusive, but it should be remembered that its purpose is purely to enable your doctor to assist you to make the best and most appropriate decision. Sterilisation must be seen as an irreversible procedure, and therefore not only your medical history but also aspects of your social history need to be taken into account. The questions you are likely to be asked and the reasons for them are dealt with below.

DISCUSSING STERILISATION WITH YOUR PARTNER

Although sterilisation involves relatively minor surgical procedures, its consequences are significant. Anyone can ask their doctor about sterilisation and, unless you are very young – under 25 – or have no children, there is unlikely to be any reason why your request should be refused. However, there are circumstances in which your present situation could alter, and you need to consider these before making a decision.

Most people find it difficult to imagine their lives changing in any significant way, but there are some important questions you need to ask yourself, however hard they may be to answer.

* *What if my marriage/relationship breaks down?* Although you may not be able to envisage such an event, many marriages do end, even some which have seemed quite satisfactory for a

long period. If you should marry again following a marriage breakdown, you might feel quite differently about having more children with your new partner. Only the person who has the operation becomes sterilised, and it will be this partner alone who suffers the consequences of the decision should their marriage break down.

* *What if I change my mind and decide I want another child?* This can occur, and a proportion of people do express regret after sterilisation. Some people may make the decision not to have any more children for financial reasons and, even if improved financial circumstances may seem unlikely, you should consider how you might feel if you found you could afford another child. Young men and women, particularly, should think very carefully about how their situation could change in the years to come.

* *What if something happened to one or more of our children?* This is the hardest question of all, and most people will not even want to consider it. Your immediate reaction may be that you could never 'replace' your children, and would not want to try. But in practice, when a catastrophe of this sort strikes a family, many younger parents, particularly, do find that, in time, they want to have more children.

WHEN IS STERILISATION INADVISABLE?

People are more likely to experience regret if they are sterilised at a time of instability – whether emotional, financial or due to any other cause. Sterilisation done when a marriage is rocky is a frequent cause of regret. Some people think it may help to save their marriage, but it does not often do so, and if a couple splits up, one of them will be unable to have children should they find another partner.

It is not a good idea for a man to undergo a vasectomy when his partner is pregnant in case something goes wrong with the pregnancy. It is also unwise for either partner to be sterilised soon after an abortion or the stillbirth of a child, when they are likely to be emotionally upset.

Occasionally, a couple may have an unsatisfactory sex life because one or both of them are worried about pregnancy, and in these cases sterilisation may help. However, sexual problems are not often cured by this means, as they usually have a deeper emotional cause.

WHICH PARTNER SHOULD BE STERILISED?

Although in most cases there is no medical reason why one partner should be sterilised rather than the other, tubal ligation is normally done under a general anaesthetic and it therefore does involve a risk which, although small, needs to be taken into account. The local anaesthetic normally used for vasectomy operations carries no equivalent risk. Although the operation is a more serious one for women than for men, it is surprising how many men do not wish to have it done.

The fallopian tubes which are cut or tied off during tubal ligation are inside the woman's body, whereas the vasa deferentia of men are more easily reached, being on the outside of the body in the scrotum. The operation for a woman is therefore more invasive. However, the reverse side of the coin is that a woman in her forties may be unlikely to have any more children, whereas a man of this age following a marriage breakdown could remarry a younger woman who may wish to have a family.

Female sterilisation is effective almost immediately after the operation, or at least after the next menstrual period. For men, sperm are still present within the remaining portions of the vasa deferentia following vasectomy, and these need to be ejected during sexual activity. The process takes about 12 to 30 ejaculations, during which time another contraceptive method must be used. Men are therefore normally asked to produce two semen samples, three and four months after their operation, to make sure that all the sperm have been ejected. The two semen samples must both be sperm free before sterilisation can be assured. This method of checking means that male sterilisation tends to be more reliable than female sterilisation, for which there is no equivalent check. However, it is still possible for vasectomies to fail, even after the production of two sperm-free samples, as occasionally the cut ends of a vas deferens can spontaneously rejoin.

If a woman does become pregnant after sterilisation, there is a signficantly increased risk of the fertilised egg implanting in a fallopian tube rather than in the uterus. Such ectopic pregnancies are dangerous for the woman, and her baby cannot survive. If an ectopic pregnancy does occur, the fallopian tube and the fetus it contains will have to be removed in an operation known as **salpingectomy**.

Reports of an increased occurrence of heart disease and testicular and prostate cancer in men who have had a vasectomy have not been substantiated, and the latest research shows no evidence of any such relationship.

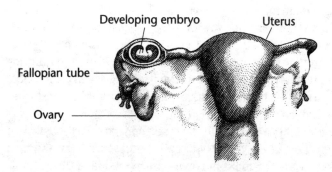

Ectopic pregnancy. This diagram shows an embryo developing from a fertilised egg which has implanted in the wall of a fallopian tube.

VISITING YOUR DOCTOR

Assuming you have talked things through with your partner, and have decided that sterilisation may be the answer for one of you, you should make an appointment to see your GP or a doctor at a family planning clinic.

The doctor is likely to ask you why you want to be sterilised, and will probably take details of your medical and contraceptive history, as well as asking you questions about your social circumstances.

You will probably be asked about your children – their ages and how they were born – and for details of your physical health. Particular emphasis will be placed on a woman's gynaecological history. Tubal ligation can be a more difficult operation to perform for women who have had pelvic **adhesions** – the sticking together of organs within the pelvic cavity – or repeated caesarean sections. For these women, the more invasive operation of laparotomy (see p.68) may be necessary rather than laparoscopy (see p.62). Unlike laparoscopy, which involves making two small incisions in the abdomen, a long incision is needed for laparotomy so that the surgeon can explore the abdominal and pelvic cavities.

If a woman suffers from heavy or painful periods, or from premenstrual tension, her doctor may suggest she has another operation, such as a hysterectomy, or takes medication. Hysterectomy involves the removal of the uterus, thus putting an end to the menstrual periods and making pregnancy impossible. However, it is major surgery and would not be considered solely as a means of contraception.

For a man who is considering vasectomy, the doctor will want to know if he has any history of undescended testicles or hernia repair as these can make the operation more difficult.

The doctor may ask you about your sex life and your feelings for each other. These questions are only to try to make sure you are considering sterilisation for appropriate reasons and are not attempting to put right problems which the operation is unlikely to solve.

Your doctor may mention alternative forms of contraception to you to make sure you have considered all your options. Many women choose sterilisation rather than continue taking the contraceptive pill long term and risk any possible side-effects it may have. As already mentioned, the general anaesthetic used to perform tubal ligation carries its own risk, albeit a small one.

Women will be asked whether there is any possibility of them being pregnant. If you have any doubts at all, it is important that you tell your doctor about them. If you are taking a contraceptive pill and are sure that you have not missed any tablets, it will be assumed that you are not pregnant. If you have not recently had a normal period, your doctor may want to do a pregnancy test before you go into hospital.

If your doctor feels that you may have some doubts about being sterilised, it may be suggested that you think things through and discuss them further with your partner before returning for another appointment. If you are less than certain yourself, you should also ask for time to consider things.

PHYSICAL EXAMINATIONS

Once the doctor is satisfied that you are happy with your decision, the partner to be sterilised will probably be examined.

Examinations for men

For men, all that is likely to be necessary is a simple examination to make sure that the external genitalia feel healthy and that surgery will be straightforward.

You will probably be asked to remove your trousers and underpants, and the doctor will gently examine your scrotum.

Each testis and vas deferens will be felt separately to check that they are mobile and not unduly tender. The presence of an infection or a tumour, or any other problem which is likely to make surgery more complicated, can usually be detected in this way.

Examinations for women

Women will probably be given a vaginal examination and possibly a cervical smear (see p.30). These are done to look for any

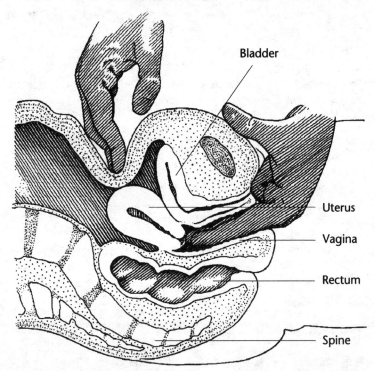

Bimanual vaginal examination. The doctor inserts two fingers into the vagina to touch the cervix. With the other hand pressing on the abdomen, the top of the uterus can be felt, and an idea obtained of its size and mobility.

other possible problems, such as ovarian cysts, which could be dealt with at the same time as the sterilisation operation.

Vaginal examination

Also known as a **bimanual examination**, this involves the doctor inserting one or two fingers into the vagina to feel the cervix. At the same time, the doctor's other hand presses down on the surface of the lower abdomen to try to feel the top of the uterus and thus to assess its size, shape, mobility and position. If the ovaries are enlarged, they too may be felt.

A further examination using a **speculum** may also be carried out. The speculum is lubricated and inserted into the vagina to stretch its walls and allow the doctor to see the cervix.

These examinations are uncomfortable but should not be painful.

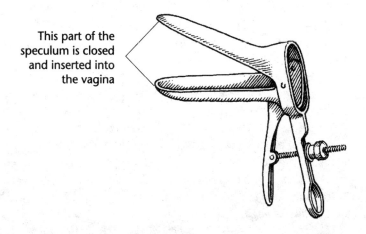

This part of the speculum is closed and inserted into the vagina

A speculum. The blades of the speculum are closed and inserted into the vagina. They are then opened as much as possible without causing undue discomfort, thus separating the walls of the vagina and allowing the doctor a clear view of the cervix.

Cervical smear

A speculum is inserted into the vagina and a specially shaped wooden spatula is rotated gently against the skin at the lower end of the cervix to remove a small sample of cells. The cells are then spread onto a microscopy slide, fixed with a chemical, and sent to a laboratory for examination under a microscope.

Cervical smears are done to detect the presence of pre-malignant changes in the cells of the cervix which, if untreated, may progress to cervical cancer. These changes can be successfully treated by the removal of a small piece of the skin from the cervix.

VISITING THE CONSULTANT

Once you and your doctor agree as to the best plan of action, you may be referred to a consultant – a gynaecologist if the woman is to be sterilised, or a urological or general surgeon if the man is to have a vasectomy and needs to be examined for any reason (see p.21). In some areas, vasectomies are not done at a hospital but at a GP's surgery which is visited by a surgeon or by a GP specially trained to carry out these operations. They can also be carried out at a family planning clinic.

If your doctor arranges for you to see a consultant, you may have to wait some time for your appointment. Sterilisation is not an urgent operation, and if the consultant has a long waiting list for more serious surgery, you will not be given priority.

Most of the questions your doctor asked you may be repeated by the consultant, perhaps with a slightly different emphasis as the consultant has probably not met you before whereas your doctor probably has.

The letter the consultant receives from your doctor will highlight any areas of concern, for example if you are young, have only one or no children, or are considering sterilisation for financial reasons rather than because you have a personal desire not to have any more children.

Again, it is a good idea for a couple to talk to the consultant together, partly because this shows that they are both agreed in their desire for sterilisation.

The consultant may repeat the vaginal or scrotal examinations described above.

Once sterilisation has been agreed upon, you may be given written details of what the operation involves and, for men, of the post-operative sperm checks and how to perform them.

The consultant should also explain any possible problems which may be encountered. For example, if laparoscopic tubal ligation is planned, there is a possibility that a laparotomy will turn out to be necessary instead when the time comes, and you should be warned about this. The recovery period following a laparotomy is longer than that for a laparoscopic operation, and there may be more discomfort from the larger wound, which will take longer to heal.

The consultant should also explain that, for women who have been taking a contraceptive pill, and therefore have had artificially light periods, menstrual bleeding may become heavier following sterilisation. If you have used a coil, your periods are likely to be lighter post-operatively, and to be much the same if a barrier method, or no contraception, was your previous choice.

You will be sent a letter from the hospital or clinic when an appointment can be made for you. Again, the length of time people have to wait for sterilisation operations varies from area to area, and can be several months at least as the operation is not essential for health reasons. If you are keen to avoid a long wait, you may want to discuss with your doctor the possibility of having your operation done privately (see Chapter 10). At family planning clinics, where sterilisation is the only type of surgery undertaken, waiting times may be shorter than at a hospital.

The consultant may ask you to sign a consent form at this stage, but this is more commonly done when you are admitted to hospital for your operation. The consent forms differ from those used for other types of surgery, and include a statement to confirm that you have been told that sterilisation does have an associated failure rate and cannot be considered to be reversible. You should read the form carefully before you sign it, and ask for an explanation of anything you do not understand.

EXAMINATION BY STUDENT DOCTORS

You may be asked if a student doctor can examine you at your out-patients' appointment or just before your operation begins. For women this may mean while they are under general anaesthetic. Only one student is permitted to carry out a vaginal examination of a woman who is under anaesthetic, and the woman's consent is always obtained beforehand, either in writing or verbally, depending on the hospital's policy. The student will perform a vaginal examination and possibly also a speculum examination.

It is very important that student doctors are able to do these examinations, both on patients who are awake and on women who are anaesthetised. It is less embarrassing for the women and the students if it is done under anaesthesia. It is also easier for the student to learn if the examination is carried out when the woman's muscles are relaxed.

If you are being treated in a teaching hospital, you are almost certain to be asked, and may be approached if you are in a district hospital which is attended by medical students. However, you can, of course, refuse your permission if you prefer; the decision is yours entirely and will not affect your treatment in any way.

REVERSAL OF STERILISATION

Both your GP and the consultant are likely to talk in detail to you about the fact that a sterilisation operation – whether for a man or woman – needs to be regarded as being permanent and irreversible. Although modern surgical techniques do make it possible to reverse the operation, success cannot be guaranteed, particularly for men and for anyone whose sterilisation operation was done more than about ten years ago. However, unlike sterilisation itself, reversal is not a minor procedure but involves major surgery with a higher incidence of complications.

It has recently become increasingly difficult to get a reversal performed under the NHS except in exceptional circumstances such as following the death of children through accident.

Reversal of tubal ligation

Before agreeing to attempt reversal of sterilisation, a laparoscopy may have to be done to look at the fallopian tubes and to discover what method of tubal ligation was used. If, following this laparoscopic examination, the doctor feels there is a reasonable chance of reversal being successful, laparotomy will be necessary. This involves making quite a large transverse incision in the lower abdomen, cutting out the ring or clip, and then cutting the fallopian tubes back to remove all the unhealthy tissue. Very small, non-absorbable stitches will then have to be used to link the two ends of each fallopian tube without closing the lumen or allowing stitches to pass through the wall of the tube into its lumen. A foreign body such as a piece of suture material within a fallopian tube can result in an ectopic pregnancy. The operation is complex, can take three to four hours to perform, and should always be done by a surgeon who has specific experience in this field.

Following a reversal operation, it is necessary to have a course of antibiotics and sometimes steroids to try to prevent adhesion of the external surface of the fallopian tubes to other organs, or of the inner surfaces of a tube to each other, which would effectively close the fallopian tube off, rendering you sterile again.

Reversal of vasectomy

Reversal of vasectomy is usually performed under general anaesthesia as a day-case procedure. Most surgeons prefer to rejoin the vasa deferentia on both sides during the same operation. Surgery takes about one to one and a half hours to perform, and recovery is similar to that following a vasectomy done under general anaesthesia.

FAILURE OF STERILISATION

Sterilisation does have a failure rate, of approximately one to four in every thousand operations performed. The failure rate is higher for women if tubal ligation is performed immediately after the birth of a child or after termination of a pregnancy. During pregnancy the fallopian tubes are enlarged and when they shrink again the clips or rings placed around them become loose. Sterilisation used to be common practice at these times, but due to the higher failure rate and incidence of regret experienced by the women concerned, it is now rare.

Failure of tubal ligation

Sterilisation may fail if the rings or clips are placed on the wrong structure, although this occurs rarely. A much more common reason for failure is that the ring or clip does not completely close off the fallopian tube and a minute passageway remains (much too small to be seen by the naked eye), allowing penetration by a sperm. It is also possible for the operation to be performed successfully but for there to be recanalisation at a later date. This occurs if there is spontaneous repair of the damage to the fallopian tubes, the severed ends of which may rejoin.

Failure of vasectomy

For men, a very rare cause of primary failure of a vasectomy is ligation of a structure other than the vas deferens, although this is an unlikely mistake for an experienced surgeon to make. Secondary failure may be due to the spontaneous repair of a vas deferens occurring after two sperm-free samples of semen have been produced. In both these cases, the failure is only detected when the man's partner becomes pregnant.

Another cause of vasectomy failure, which may occur in about 2 per cent of cases, is the presence of **lurking sperm**. Where these occur, the semen samples are never completely clear, although they may contain only *very* small numbers of non-motile sperm. Although there is very little risk of the man's partner becoming pregnant, the operation is usually repeated under general anaesthetic, which invariably resolves the problem.

CHAPTER 4

Going in to hospital

This chapter deals mainly with what is likely to happen if you are admitted to hospital for a vasectomy or tubal ligation involving the use of a general anaesthetic. Although you may stay in hospital overnight after your operation, or possibly for two or three nights if you are having a laparotomy, day-case surgery is also discussed here as it is now a common way of dealing with sterilisation operations.

The majority of vasectomy operations are done using a local anaesthetic and normally involve less than an hour at a vasectomy clinic. You will probably be asked to shave and wash your scrotal area carefully before you attend for your appointment. You may need to take with you slippers and a dressing gown, as in some hospitals you will be required to walk to the operating theatre rather than being taken on a trolley. Some money for the telephone and something to read while you are waiting may also be a good idea. It is best to wear close-fitting underpants after a vasectomy to help support the scrotum.

If you are staying in hospital overnight, items 2 to 10 in the list on pp.42–43 may be useful.

Local anaesthesia for tubal ligation is rarely available under the NHS. If you are having this operation at a private clinic, you will probably be sent all the necessary information beforehand.

Whatever the arrangements are for your operation, you will probably receive a letter from the hospital telling you the date of your appointment and any other details you need to know. Many hospitals also send out leaflets explaining the admission procedures and advising you what to take in with you. You may have been put on a shortlist so that if an unexpected gap occurs in the operating schedule, you will be asked to come in at short notice – possibly within a day or two.

DAY-CASE SURGERY

Sterilisation involving the use of general anaesthesia is now normally done as day-case surgery for people who are fit and healthy.

The average cost of an operation involving an overnight stay in hospital is approximately three to four times greater than the cost of the operation done as a day case. Now that hospital expenditure is a major consideration, day-case surgery is seen as a sensible way of cutting costs and reducing the length of waiting lists.

You will be admitted to hospital at least an hour or two before your operation and will leave again within a few hours, once you have recovered from the anaesthetic. Patients have to be screened very carefully to make sure that only those whose general health is good are selected for this type of care. You may therefore be asked to attend a pre-admission clerking clinic for tests to detect any problems which may make you unsuitable for day-case surgery or which would alert medical staff to the need for any special precautions to be taken during your treatment.

As anyone having a general anaesthetic should be looked after by a responsible adult overnight after their operation, single parents caring for children or those living only with a disabled adult, for example, will have to make suitable arrangements. However, a request to stay overnight in hospital if you have any problems is likely to be sympathetically considered. It is a good idea to have made plans for children to be cared for, for example, in the event that a minor complication occurs and you have to stay overnight in hospital after your operation.

HOSPITAL STAFF

The ward of a hospital is a busy place and can seem rather confusing and frightening. It may help to have an idea of the different medical staff you are likely to meet, and the jobs they do.

Nurses

The uniforms worn to distinguish nurses of different ranks will vary from hospital to hospital. In some hospitals, the nurses all wear the same uniform, but with their grades indicated by, for example, belts of different colours. All nurses wear badges which state clearly their name and sometimes their grade. There are, of course, both male and female nurses, although women are still in the majority. The nursing grades are as follows.

1   The most senior nurse on the ward is the *ward sister* or *ward manager*. Each ward will have one ward sister who will be very experienced and able to answer any questions you may have. The ward sister has 24-hour a day responsibility for all the staff and patients on at least one ward, for the day-to-day running of the ward, standards of care etc., and is ultimately responsible for the ward even when not on duty. The ward sister will be a registered nurse (RN), who has usually been qualified for at least five years. Ward sisters may wear a uniform of a single colour, often dark blue.

   The male equivalent of the ward sister is a *charge nurse*. Charge nurses often wear a white tunic.

2   When the ward sister is not on duty, there may be a *senior staff nurse* in charge. The senior staff nurse is deputy to, and works closely with, the ward sister. Like the ward sister, this nurse will be very experienced.

3   Each ward may have several *staff nurses*. These are registered nurses who have completed their nursing training. They may

be newly qualified or may have several years' experience, and will take charge of the ward when both the ward sister and senior staff nurse are unavailable. There are different grades of staff nurse, each distinguished by a different coloured belt, hat or uniform.

The more junior staff nurses are very often in their first or second post since qualifying. They are less involved in ward management, and are therefore able to work closely with the patients. Most of the staff nurses on a ward will be junior staff nurses.

4   *Enrolled nurses* are gradually being replaced. They have undergone two years of training and, like the junior staff nurses, are mainly involved in patient care rather than ward management.

5   As student nurses now spend more time in college and less on the wards of hospitals, *health care assistants* (HCAs) have been brought in to take their place. These are unqualified nurses who have undergone six months' training on day release while working on a ward and who have then been assessed for a National Vocational Qualification by senior nurses. Health care assistants are able to carry out all basic nursing duties except for the dispensing of drugs. They are supervised at all times by a qualified nurse.

6   The ward may also have several *nursing auxiliaries*. These are not trained nurses, but are present on the ward to deal with any non-medical jobs and to help with the basic care of patients. Their duties include making beds, handing out tea, and putting away linen etc.

7   Student nurses – *diploma nursing students* or *Project 2000 students* – are unpaid, and allocated to the wards at various stages during their college-based training. They are mainly involved in observing, and carrying out limited clinical tasks. In their last term before they qualify, they will be rostered on to nursing shifts and be part of a ward team.

Doctors

Each consultant surgeon in a hospital heads a team of doctors of different ranks, sometimes known as a 'firm'. You may meet some or all of them. These doctors can, of course, be men or women.

1   The *consultant surgeon* holds the ultimate responsibility for all the patients on the operating list, and for the work of all the staff in the 'firm'. Consultants have at least 10 to 15 years' experience as surgeons.

    You may never actually see the consultant surgeon who is responsible for your care, but you may be visited on the ward before your operation by whichever surgeon is to perform it.

2   The *senior registrar* is a very experienced surgeon who has completed several years of training and will soon be appointed to a consultant's post.

3   *Registrars* have trained as surgeons for at least two or three years and are able to carry out some surgery alone, assisting the consultant, or being assisted by the consultant, on more difficult operations.

4   Some hospitals employ *clinical assistants* as surgeons. These are often very experienced surgeons who, for personal or family reasons, are not able to work full time. You may not meet this surgeon before your operation.

5   Before your operation you may be examined on the ward by a *senior house officer* (SHO), or by a house surgeon (see below). Senior house officers have been qualified doctors for between one and five years, and are gaining further experience in hospital before becoming surgeons or specialising in another branch of medicine.

6   A *house surgeon* (or *house officer*) may be directly concerned with your care both before and after your operation, taking notes of your medical history and arranging for any

necessary pre-operative investigations to be done, such as a blood count, chest X-ray or electrocardiogram. House officers are qualified doctors who have completed at least five years of undergraduate training and are working for a further year in hospital before becoming fully registered doctors. Although house officers do not perform surgery on their own, they may assist the surgeon in the operating theatre.

Anaesthetists

Anaesthetists are highly trained doctors who specialise in giving anaesthetics and in pain relief. An anaesthetist will also visit you before your operation to discuss any relevant details, such as any anaesthetics you have had in the past and any drugs you may be taking (see Chapter 5).

OPERATIONS INVOLVING A GENERAL ANAESTHETIC

Length of stay in hospital

Vasectomy

If you do have to stay overnight in hospital after a vasectomy, you are likely to be discharged the following day when you have recovered from the general anaesthetic and are fit to care for yourself. Otherwise you will be able to leave within a few hours, at most.

Tubal ligation

Unless you are being treated as a day case (see p.37), you will probably only have to spend one night in hospital following a laparoscopic tubal ligation, and possibly two or three nights if you have a laparotomy. Even if laparoscopy is planned, it is best to be prepared to spend longer in hospital in case laparotomy is found to be necessary once surgery begins, for the reasons mentioned on p.70. This possibility will be discussed with you beforehand.

What to take into hospital with you

Tubal ligation
As you are unlikely to be in hospital for longer than two or three days, at most, you will not need to take much in with you. The following list may be helpful.

1 *Sanitary pads.* Although the hospital will probably provide you with sanitary pads for use immediately after your operation, those issued by hospitals are likely to be the old-fashioned type, and many women prefer to use the ones they are used to. It is expensive for hospitals to supply sanitary pads and therefore women are usually encouraged to provide their own whenever possible. Sanitary pads are necessary because of the small amount of vaginal bleeding which often occurs during the first day or two after surgery.
2 *Nightclothes.* You will be given a hospital shift to wear during the operation itself, but many people prefer to put on their own nightclothes as soon as possible afterwards. If you stay in hospital overnight, or longer, you will need your own.
3 *Slippers.*
4 *Dressing gown.*
5 *Towel and washing things.*
6 *Money.* A small amount of money may be useful for newspapers and the telephone. Large sums of money, wallets and handbags should not be taken into hospital as these may have to be kept in an unlocked cabinet by your bed. If you do have to take any valuables or large sums of money into hospital, you should give these to the nurse in charge of your ward when you are admitted. You will be given a receipt listing each item and this should be kept

safe so that you can collect your possessions when you are discharged. However, hospital authorities strongly discourage people from bringing anything of great value with them unless absolutely necessary.

7 *Books and magazines*. There will inevitably be periods of waiting between visits from medical staff before your operation, and you may want something to occupy you during this time, as well as during your post-operative stay.

8 *Loose clothing and shoes*. Clothes such as tight jeans will be uncomfortable after your operation. Casual, comfortable jogging trousers, or similar, are ideal.

9 *Drugs you are already taking*. Once your admission has been arranged, your GP will have been asked to fill in a form stating all the drugs you are taking and their doses. You may also be asked to take your drugs with you when you go into hospital so that their dosages can be checked and so that you can continue to be given any which are necessary. All your drugs will be kept for you during your stay as you must only take those which are given to you by medical staff. If you are asked to take your own drugs into hospital, these should be returned to you before you leave.

10 *Admission letter*. An admission letter will have been sent to you from the hospital, and you should take this with you when you are admitted for your operation.

Jewellery

Whenever possible, all jewellery should be left at home. Although wedding rings may be worn during an operation, there is a risk that any jewellery you take off before surgery may be lost or stolen. If you have to take any jewellery into hospital, it should be given to the ward sister for safe keeping.

BLEEDING DURING SURGERY IS CONTROLLED BY **electro-cautery**. An electric current is used to heat the tip of an instrument which then shrivels and seals the little blood vessels and stops the bleeding. Therefore wedding rings, or any other rings which are very precious to you or which cannot be removed, will be covered with adhesive tape during surgery as metal can cause electrical burns or electric shocks during this process.

Procedures before the operation

Admission to the ward

When you arrive at the hospital, you should report to the main reception desk with your admission letter. The staff there will check your details and tell you which ward to go to. Once on the ward, the ward clerk will deal with the clerical side of your admission, filling in the necessary forms with you. If you are staying in hospital overnight, you will then be allocated a bed and introduced to your **named nurse** who will look after you during your stay.

The Named Nurse Initiative was introduced into NHS hospitals under the Government's Patients' Charter. A particular nurse is now responsible for planning each patient's nursing care throughout their stay in hospital. (The ward sister will, of course, still be informed of all aspects of your care, and will be able to discuss it with you or your relatives.)

Do tell the nurse if you have any problems or if you are anxious about *any* aspect of your hospital stay.

As you are admitted to the ward, the nurse will take notes of your personal details and explain the ward procedures to you. Your discharge will also be planned at this time. The nursing staff will need to be sure that someone will be able to collect you and take you home when the time comes. Before you are due to go home, the nurses will have to be sure you can manage. The anaesthetic gases, and other agents used by the anaesthetist, can stay in your body for several days, and although you may feel you are fully recovered, your reaction times may be slow and you may continue to feel sick and light-headed for at least the next couple of days.

The nurse will measure your blood pressure, temperature and pulse. A sample of your urine may be taken for analysis to make sure you do not have diabetes or any disorder of the kidneys which would make the operation inadvisable. You may also be weighed as the anaesthetist may need to know your weight in order to be able to calculate the dose of anaesthetic you require.

Visit by the house surgeon or senior house officer

As has already been mentioned, a house surgeon or senior house officer may visit you on the ward before your operation to take details of your medical history, including any allergies you have and any drugs you are taking, and to examine you. Your GP may have already filled in a form giving the names and dosages of any drugs you have been prescribed, and you should have been told what to do about these. Do not forget to tell the hospital doctor of any other drugs you have been taking which your GP may not be aware of, such as vitamin supplements, cough medicines, aspirins etc., which are available from the chemist without the need for prescription.

Women who normally take contraceptive pills should not stop these before their operation. It may be possible to stop taking them immediately after your operation, but you are likely to be told to finish your current packet before doing so.

A medical examination is carried out to identify any illness or infection you may have which could complicate the use of a general anaesthetic. Investigations such as a chest X-ray and electrocardiogram may be requested if you suffer from asthma, unexplained fainting, or are a heavy smoker.

The house surgeon will probably also ask you to sign a consent form if you have not already done so. Although it can be assumed that your consent to the operation is implied by the fact that you have entered hospital willingly, consent forms are widely used. By signing this form you are declaring that your operation has been explained to you and that you understand what it entails and have agreed to it taking place. You are also giving your permission for the doctors to take whatever action they feel to be appropriate should some emergency occur during your operation, and for any necessary anaesthetic to be given to you. Do read this form carefully, and ask the doctor to explain anything you do not understand.

Visit by the surgeon

The surgeon who is to perform your operation may also visit you on the ward to check that all is well.

Visit by the anaesthetist

The anaesthetist will probably come to see you to ask you about anything that may be relevant to the choice of anaesthetic given to you.

Anaesthetics have improved considerably during the last few years, and a 'pre-med.' is now not always given routinely. If you or your anaesthetist do feel that you are very anxious and need something to relax you, you may be given some form of sedative, by mouth or injection, one or two hours before the operation.

If you have any false teeth, crowns or dental bridges, you should tell the anaesthetist. False teeth will have to be removed before you go into the operating theatre.

'Nil by mouth'

This is a term which means that neither food nor drink must be swallowed. In order to prevent vomiting and the risk of choking on your vomit while you are anaesthetised, you will be told not to eat or drink anything for about six hours before your operation, although you will be able to have a few sips of water with any tablets you need to take.

Shaving
Before undergoing a vasectomy, the scrotum must be shaved and carefully washed. This can be done at home the day before your operation, or at the hospital once you have been admitted to the ward. Shaving is not necessary prior to tubal ligation.

Anti-embolism stockings
If you are having a laparotomy, once you are settled on the ward a nurse may measure your legs for **T**hrombo-**E**mbolic **D**eterrent **S**tockings (TEDS) to wear during your operation. These stockings used to be worn only by patients having major operations to help prevent blood clots forming in the veins deep within the legs as they lay motionless on the operating table, sometimes for several hours. However, they are now used routinely as a precaution in many operations, including laparotomy for tubal ligation. Although they may feel uncomfortable, particularly when the weather is hot, there is no doubt as to their value.

The normal activity of the muscles in the legs helps to keep the blood moving through them. During long periods of bed rest or anaesthesia, these muscles are inactive and the circulation of blood in the legs slows down. A blood clot is thus more likely to form which can block the passage of blood through the vein. If pieces of this clot break off, they form **emboli**. Even one embolus may have serious consequences if it travels through the circulation and lodges in a vital organ such as the lung. Anti-embolism stockings improve the return of venous blood to the heart and thus help to prevent blood clots forming.

If you are to be given TEDS, the nurse will measure your calf and thigh and the length of your leg, and will give you a pair of stockings of the correct size. If you have a history of varicose veins or thrombosis which increases your risk of developing a blood clot, it is probably important to wear the stockings throughout your hospital stay.

SMOKING

If you are a heavy smoker and have not been able to cut down or stop altogether, you will be advised not to smoke in the hours before your operation. It is, of course, much better to stop smoking some months before surgery. The carbon monoxide contained in cigarette smoke poisons the blood by replacing some of the oxygen which is carried in it and which is vital to processes such as wound healing.

OBESITY

Obesity also adds to the risk of anaesthesia, and for this reason people who are very overweight should try to lose weight before entering hospital. Indeed, some surgeons will not carry out non-emergency operations on heavy smokers or obese patients as they consider the risks to be too great. However, starting a long, strict diet before your operation may also be inadvisable. The consultant will have assessed your weight when seeing you at your out-patients' appointment, and will probably have given you some guidance at that time.

Obese women will probably be warned that although laparoscopy may be attempted, the surgeon is likely to have to revert to laparotomy if the laparoscope cannot be inserted through the bulk of fatty tissue.

WAITING

It may seem that you have been admitted to hospital unnecessarily early, and you may find you have to wait on the ward with little to do. Apart from having to be seen by the medical staff mentioned above, who are responsible for many other patients as well, time will also have been allowed for the assessment of any medical problems you may have, and for the results of any blood tests to be received.

Sometimes operations are cancelled at the last moment. Although this is distressing, and can be very awkward for someone who has had to make special arrangements to come into hospital, it only occurs if an emergency has arisen. If your operation does have to be cancelled, another appointment will be made for you as soon as possible.

You will probably be given only an approximate time for your operation, and be told if it is scheduled for the morning or afternoon. An operation being done before yours may take longer than expected if complications arise.

LEAVING THE WARD FOR YOUR OPERATION

Before being taken from the ward to the anaesthetic room or operating theatre, you will be given a hospital operating gown to wear and, if relevant, will be asked to put on your anti-embolism stockings. A plastic-covered bracelet bearing your name and an identifying hospital number will be attached to one or both of your wrists. You will then probably be taken from the ward on a hospital trolley. A nurse from the ward will accompany you to the anaesthetic room so that you have with you someone you recognise and who knows a little about you.

CHAPTER 5

Anaesthesia

LOCAL ANAESTHESIA

Vasectomy

As has already been mentioned, vasectomies are usually done under local anaesthetic, although general anaesthesia may be necessary for men who have had previous surgery to repair a hernia or undescended testicles, or certain infections (see p.21). General anaesthesia can also be used for men who have an allergy to local anaesthetic, and it may be possible for those who would simply prefer it. You are likely to have to wait longer before an operation can be done under a general anaesthetic.

If you have a strong preference, or know that you are allergic to any type of anaesthetic, you should mention this to your doctor, or consultant if you see one.

When you are called into the operating room, you will be asked to lie on your back on the operating table, and the local anaesthetic will be injected directly into your scrotum over the area where the surgeon will make an incision. The anaesthetic takes effect almost immediately, causing complete loss of painful sensation at the site of the planned incision in the scrotum, and will continue to act for up to six hours.

The needle used to inject the anaesthetic is of a smaller diameter than that used for taking blood, and although the anaesthetic will sting slightly as it enters your body, the injection should not be too uncomfortable.

Unlike a general anaesthetic, a local anaesethetic does not cause drowsiness or nausea after the operation.

Tubal ligation

It is possible for tubal ligation to be performed using a local anaesthetic, but this method is not normally available at NHS hospitals. It is, however, available privately at the Elliot Smith Clinic in the Churchill Hospital, Oxford, and at the Margaret Pike Clinic in London. It may also be practised at large family planning clinics in the future. Laparoscopic tubal ligation done with a local anaesthetic involves a stay at the clinic of about two hours. The anaesthetic itself is injected through the ports inserted in the small incisions made in the abdomen (see p.65), and a sedative and painkiller are injected into a vein in the back of the hand.

GENERAL ANAESTHESIA

The information given in this section applies to women undergoing tubal ligation, as well as to men whose vasectomies are to be carried out under general anaesthetic.

Most sterilisation operations for women are now done as day-case surgery (see p.37). You may be admitted to a special day-case ward at the hospital on the day of your operation, where you are likey to be visited by an anaesthetist as well as by a doctor on the surgical team. An anaesthetist is a hospital doctor who has been trained in the special skills of giving drugs which cause loss of sensation or consciousness, or both (anaesthetics), and those which block feelings of pain (analgesics). Anaesthesia is a vital part of any operation, and a great deal of time and trouble will be taken to make sure that you receive the anaesthetic which best suits you.

The main reason for the anaesthetist's visit before your operation is to decide what type of anaesthesia would be safest for you. It also gives you the opportunity to discuss any problems or worries you may have concerning your anaesthesia.

The anaesthetist will ask you several questions about any anaesthetics you have had before, any drugs you are taking, and about your general health. It is important that you answer these questions as fully as possible. The anaesthetist will want to know if you have any crowned or capped teeth as these may require special attention. You should also mention if you have false teeth, as they will have to be removed before your operation to avoid them being inhaled into your lungs while you are anaesthetised.

If you have had any problems in the past such as an allergy to a particular anaesthetic, it will be helpful if you know the name of the drug concerned or the hospital where the operation was carried out. The appropriate records can then be checked to make sure another type of anaesthetic is used for your sterilisation operation. You should also tell the anaesthetist if you know of any other member of your family who has had a problem with any type of anaesthesia, as it is possible that you may have the same reaction to a particular drug.

The anaesthetist may also want to examine you and to look at the results of any tests you have had.

The drugs used will put you to sleep so that you have no feeling in any part of your body. General anaesthetics can be given in two different ways.

1   *Intravenous anaesthetic.* A general anaesthetic of this type can be injected into a vein via a plastic tube which is inserted into your hand or arm. It will put you to sleep within a few seconds.
2   *Inhalational anaesthetic.* This is a gas which you breathe in through a face mask. It acts within one to two minutes. As some people find the use of a face mask alarming, it is not normally applied until you are asleep.

During the operation, the anaesthetist will make sure you stay asleep by giving you more drugs as necessary.

You will have been told not to have anything to eat or drink for at least six hours before surgery ('nil by mouth'). The reason for this is that any food or drink left in your stomach when you are anaesthetised could cause you to be sick during the operation.

While you are still on the ward, you will be given any medicines you normally take, such as diuretics ('water tablets') or drugs to reduce high blood pressure. Pre-medication ('premed.') is not normally given before sterilisation operations.

You will then be taken from the ward, probably on a hospital trolley, to the anaesthetic room or straight into the operating theatre to be given your anaesthetic.

The anaesthetist, or an assistant, will ask you several questions to confirm your identity and make sure that you are the right person for the operation. Your identity bands will also be checked. Many people have many types of operations each day in a hospital, and these checks, which may be repeated, are essential to make sure no mistakes are made.

The anaesthetist will then fit various monitoring devices to watch over you while you are asleep. A probe may be attached to your finger to measure the amount of oxygen in your blood; some sticky pads may be put on your chest so that your heart beat can be recorded on an electrocardiograph; and a cuff may be put around your arm to measure your blood pressure. All these monitoring devices enable the anaesthetist to make sure that the anaesthetic remains effective and that you remain well during surgery.

A plastic cannula will be put into a vein in the back of your hand or arm, and the anaesthetic drugs will be introduced into your body through this.

Once the anaesthetist is happy with the readings from the monitors, your anaesthesia can start. The anaesthetist will remain with you throughout your operation, and will still be there when you wake up.

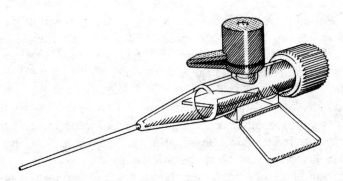

A butterfly cannula. A commonly used type of cannula through which drugs can be injected into a vein (usually in the back of the hand) during an operation.

The anaesthetic

Once the anaesthetic has been injected, you will fall asleep within seconds. The drug which makes you go to sleep may sting a little as it enters the vein from the cannula, but this feeling does not last long. Instead of an injection, you may be asked to breathe a sweet-smelling gas to put you to sleep.

Several different types of drugs will be given to you to make sure you remain asleep. The following are used to anaesthetise you.

1   *Induction agents*: drugs which bring on sleep.
2   *Maintenance agents*: drugs which keep you asleep.
3   *Analgesics*: drugs which stop you feeling pain after the operation.
4   *Anti-emetics*: drugs which help to stop you feeling sick after the operation.

Local anaesthetic may also be injected into the wound during your operation to reduce the pain when you wake up and, if so, your groin may be numb for a few hours afterwards.

After your operation

When your operation is over, the anaesthetist will stop giving you the drugs that were keeping you asleep, and you will then probably be taken to a recovery room or step-down ward.

The recovery room

The nurses in the recovery room are specially trained to care for patients coming round from anaesthetics after an operation. You will stay in this room, still watched over by monitoring equipment, until you are fully awake and ready to be returned to your own ward.

If you are in pain when you wake up, tell a nurse in the recovery room as you can be given an injection or tablets to relieve this.

The step-down ward

If, as is most likely, you are going home on the same day as your operation, you may be taken to a 'step-down' ward. The nurses on this ward will make sure that you are fit to go home and that your journey will be safe and pain free. They will also want to be sure that you have a responsible adult to care for you once you are at home, and should give you advice about how to manage your recovery over the next few days.

Back on the ward

If you are not going home the same day, you will be taken back to your own ward, where the anaesthetist may visit you before you leave. This visit is to ensure that you are pain free and have no ill-effects from your operation. Do tell the anaesthetist if you have any concerns or questions.

Side-effects of general anaesthetics

There are side-effects which can occur after anaesthesia, but these do not normally last longer than a couple of days. A sore throat is quite common, and is caused by the dry gases breathed while you are asleep, or by the tube which may have been put down your throat to help you breathe during your operation. This side-effect should disappear within a few days.

When you wake up after your operation, you may have pain in the area of the wound, as well as referred pain in your shoulder if you have had a laparoscopic operation (see p.75), but if you feel unwell, or have pain other than this which causes you concern, do tell the anaesthetist – or a nurse on your ward – so that the reasons for it can be discovered.

Risks of general anaesthesia

People with certain medical conditions, such as heart or lung disease, may not be given general anaesthetics as they are potentially at greater risk.

Some people are afraid of being put to sleep by a general anaesthetic because they fear the possibility of never waking up or of suffering brain damage. Even today, with the tremendous advances that have been made in anaesthesia, risks do exist which, although small, have to be borne in mind. If you are worried about this, you should discuss with your anaesthetist the possibility of having an alternative anaesthetic.

PAIN RELIEF

The house surgeon and nurses on your ward will be able to give you analgesics to control any post-operative pain. However, if these drugs are not enough, do tell a doctor or nurse, who may be able to give you something more effective.

The amount of pain suffered after a sterilisation operation varies from person to person. Some women have pain or slight discomfort for only 12 to 24 hours and will not need any pain-killing injections. Others may need injections after their operation, possibly for up to 48 hours following laparotomy, and if so, you may have to stay in hospital overnight so that these can be given to you. In the majority of cases following laparoscopy, almost everyone is able to go home within a few hours.

CHAPTER 6

The operation: vasectomy

Vasectomy is a simple, straightforward surgical procedure which takes less than 30 minutes to perform. When, as is usually the case, it involves the use of a local anaesthetic, it can be done in an out-patients' clinic, family planning clinic, specially equipped GP's surgery, or in an operating theatre at a hospital.

When the time of your operation approaches, you will be asked to remove the clothing from your lower body, and probably to put on a dressing gown supplied for you. You can then walk into the operating room, where you will be asked to lie on the operating table on your back with your legs slightly apart. After your scrotum, penis and the upper part of your thighs have been wiped with an antiseptic solution, a sterile cloth or paper towel will be placed over the lower half of your body to keep this area clean. Your scrotum will be exposed through a hole in the cloth.

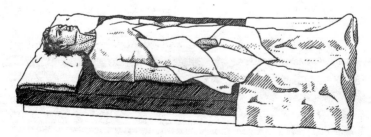

Preparing for a vasectomy. Sterile cloths are placed over the lower part of the body, leaving the penis and scrotum exposed.

Having examined your scrotum and rolled the scrotal skin between his or her fingers to identify the vas deferens on one side, the surgeon will then clasp the vas firmly between finger and thumb while injecting the local anaesthetic into the overlying skin of your scrotum. The anaesthetic will take effect almost immediately. A small incision, about 1 cm long (less than 1/2 inch), is then made in the scrotal skin directly over the vas. Some surgeons use a single midline incision, and others a small lateral one over each of the two vasa deferentia. A loop of the vas is pulled gently through the incision with specially designed forceps, and a segment, about 2 to 3 cm (approximately 1 inch) long, is cut from it. The cut ends are then tied off. Some surgeons then bury the cut ends of the vas in the tissue within the scrotum to prevent them rejoining; others double them back on themselves.

The incision in the scrotal skin will probably be closed using dissolvable stitches or small paper strips. A thin plastic film may then be sprayed over the wound, or it may be covered with a gauze swab, to be held in place by your underpants.

The whole procedure will then be repeated on the vas deferens on the other side of your scrotum.

You will be able to walk from the operating theatre to get dressed again, and should sit for a while if necessary until any feeling of faintness passes. It is advisable not to attempt to drive yourself home after this operation in case you begin to feel faint.

It is best to wear close-fitting underpants or a scrotal support for a few days to reduce the chances of bleeding and help lessen any discomfort. Apart from taking painkillers such as paracetamol to reduce your discomfort when the local anaesthetic effect wears off, an ice pack, ice cubes in a plastic bag, or a packet of frozen peas held on the scrotum may be helpful.

Further details of what to expect during your post-operative recovery are given in Chapter 8.

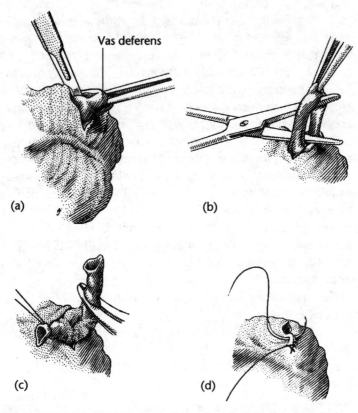

Vasectomy. (a) An incision is made in the scrotum, through which a loop of the vas deferens is gently pulled out. The loop is isolated (b), and then cut (c), and a segment of the vas is removed. The cut ends are tied off and separated. (d) The incision in the scrotum is closed using dissolvable stitches.

CHAPTER 7

The operation: tubal ligation

In its widest sense, female sterilisation includes any operation which leaves a woman unable to conceive spontaneously. It therefore encompasses the surgical removal of the womb (hysterectomy) and of the fallopian tubes (salpingectomy), as well as segmental excision and ligation of the fallopian tubes. Tubal ligation (sometimes called occlusion) is the operation most commonly performed to render a woman sterile, unless she has some other problem, such as heavy periods, which would make a hysterectomy more appropriate (see p.11), and it is therefore the method described here.

In the past, sterilisation was also carried out by **culdotomy**. This involves making an incision in the top of the vagina so that the fallopian tubes can be pulled down through the vagina and a segment of each cut away. However, there are complications associated with this operation, and it is now rarely performed.

Sterilisation operations also used to involve one of two types of **diathermy** in which an electric current was used to destroy a large portion of each fallopian tube. The operation had its drawbacks in that the bowel or abdomen could be accidentally burnt, and it was not always possible to ensure that the inner segment of the fallopian tube had been destroyed. Reversal of the procedure was more difficult.

Research is currently being carried out into the possibility of performing sterilisation operations by inserting a telescope through the cervix and into the uterus and placing a plug in each fallopian tube. Operations done in this way would not involve making any incisions at all. However, this type of surgery is still experimental, and has not so far proved very successful.

Tubal ligation can be performed using either laparoscopy or laparotomy but, whenever possible, laparoscopy is the method of choice. Rings and clips are a more expensive means of closing the fallopian tubes, and therefore are not used in laparotomy when the larger incision allows the surgeon easier access to cut and tie the tubes. Segmental excision is much more difficult to perform using the laparoscope, and is therefore rarely done when laparoscopy is the operation of choice.

LAPAROSCOPIC STERILISATION

Recent developments in the design of surgical instruments have enabled a range of operations to be performed through multiple small incisions rather than through one larger one. The linchpin of these new techniques is the laparoscope. A laparoscope is a small telescope with a video camera and a light source attached which enable the surgeon to see the organs within the abdominal cavity displayed on a television screen in the operating theatre. It is inserted into a small incision (about 1 cm across) made just below the umbilicus, and other specialised surgical instruments are inserted through another small incision made just below the pubic hairline.

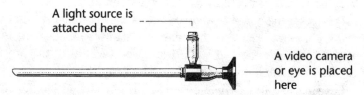

A light source is attached here

A video camera or eye is placed here

A laparoscope. The laparoscope is inserted through a small incision in the abdomen, and allows the surgeon to see into the abdominal cavity.

Laparoscopic surgery is also known as minimal access, minimally invasive or 'keyhole' surgery. It has the advantage of allowing an early discharge from hospital, usually within a few hours of the operation, and it results in less painful, smaller wounds and a more rapid return to normal activity is possible than following conventional surgery. It also gives better cosmetic results. When a laparoscope is being used, sterilisation is achieved by ligating the fallopian tubes with rings or clips. When keyhole surgery was originally done in the UK in the 1960s, it was used solely for sterilisation operations. It is therefore a tried and tested means of performing sterilisation, with which surgeons have had much experience.

The operation

Once the general anaesthetic has taken effect, you will be placed in the lithotomy position on the operating table, and your abdomen will be washed with antiseptic solution. A catheter is

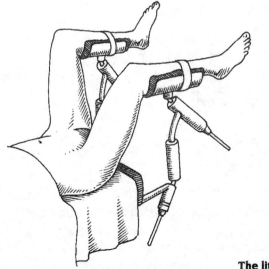

The lithotomy position.

then passed through the urethra into the bladder to empty it of its urine and thus help to ensure that it does not expand during the operation and get in the way of the operating instruments and risk being damaged.

The surgeon's assistant will perform a vaginal examination (see p.29) to assess the size and position of your uterus. A speculum can then be inserted into the vagina (see p.29) so that the cervix can be seen. The anterior lip of the cervix is grasped with a special instrument, the probe of which is inserted into the uterus. The surgeon's assistant can then use this instrument to move the uterus as required during the operation and allow the surgeon to see and reach the fallopian tubes.

The surgeon will then make a small vertical or horizontal incision either within or just below the umbilicus, through which a

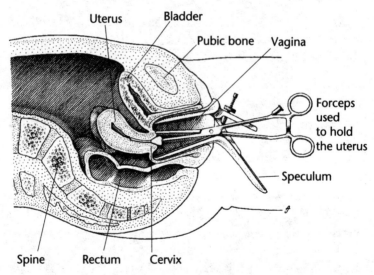

Female sterilisation. A speculum is inserted into the vagina to allow the surgeon to see the cervix. The cervix is grasped in forceps so that it can be moved during surgery, thus also moving the uterus and giving the surgeon good access to the fallopian tubes.

special needle is inserted. Carbon dioxide gas is pumped through this needle into the abdominal cavity to inflate it and allow the surgeon a clear view of the fallopian tubes as well as space in which to manipulate the surgical instruments. A special gas-delivery system ensures that the abdomen remains inflated during surgery. When used in this way, carbon dioxide is a harmless gas, and any which remains in the abdomen after the operation is absorbed by the body and expired by the lungs.

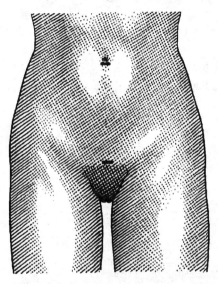

Common sites of incision for laparoscopic female sterilisation.
Each incision is approximately 1 cm long. The upper one is sometimes vertical.

Once the abdomen is sufficiently inflated, the special needle is replaced by a tube called a **trocar** or **port** which incorporates valves to allow the continued delivery of carbon dioxide and the insertion of the laparoscope. The surgeon can then see and examine the ovaries, uterus etc. for signs of any abnormality.

A similar small incision is then made in the lower abdomen and an instrument is inserted through it with which the surgeon can grasp each fallopian tube in turn. A loop of fallopian tube is pulled into the ring applicator and a ring is then pushed off the applicator onto the tube. Alternatively, a clip can be placed directly over the tube. To make sure that the rings or clips are placed on the fallopian tubes rather than on another structure (such as a ligament), the surgeon will trace each fallopian tube from its insertion into the uterus to its open end.

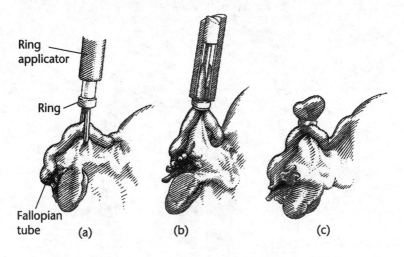

Ring applicator

Ring

Fallopian tube

(a)   (b)   (c)

Female sterilisation using a ring. (a) The fallopian tube is grasped and a loop of it is pulled up into the ring applicator. (b) The ring is pushed down over the loop of fallopian tube, which is then released from the applicator. (c) The ring closes the fallopian tube at the base of the loop, thus preventing the passage of ova within it.

When both fallopian tubes have been closed off and the operation is complete, the instruments can be withdrawn from the abdominal cavity, and the two small incisions closed using dissolvable stitches.

Clips and rings

Tubal ligation is now almost always done using clips or rings. Both are equally effective and destroy minimal amounts of tissue. Different surgeons use whichever form they are most familiar with.

Failure of a tubal ligation operation may occur if a clip is not positioned over the entire fallopian tube, or if a part of the lumen of the tube fails to be drawn into the applicator before a ring is inserted over it. Although it is possible for the ring or clip to be placed over the wrong structure, or for a fallopian tube to be torn during surgery, these are rare complications when the operation is performed by an experienced surgeon.

Rings

Several different types of rings are available (e.g. Fallope, Yoon, Ley), all of which have a basically similar design. The Fallope ring, for example, is made of silicone rubber with 5 per cent barium sulphate which enables it to be seen on X-ray. It has an outer diameter of 3.6 mm, an inner diameter of 1 mm, and it is 2.2 mm thick.

As the rings have to be stretched to load them onto the applicator, and as they must not be distorted for any longer than is necessary, loading is done just before the surgeon needs them. Once the ring has been forced off the applicator onto the narrowest part of the fallopian tube, it contracts down to its original diameter, thus effectively occluding the tube.

Clips

There are also several types of clips available (e.g. Hulka Clemens, Filshie), again all of similar design. The Filshie is approximately 1 cm long and 4 mm wide, and is made of stainless steel with a silicone rubber insert. It is introduced into the abdominal cavity on an applicator, in the same way as the Fallope ring, and is then pushed over the whole fallopian tube

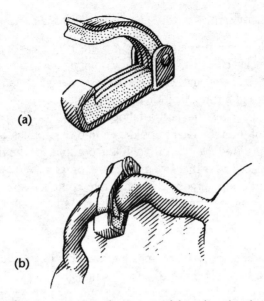

Female sterilisation using a clip. (a) A Filshie clip. (b) The clip is placed over the fallopian tube to close it.

and locked into position so that it cannot move. The silicone rubber inside the clip maintains a pressure on the fallopian tube until the portion of it which lies between the arms of the clip dies. Once this section of tissue has been destroyed, the fallopian tube becomes separated into two parts.

LAPAROTOMY

Segmental excision is done by laparotomy, and this operation is used instead of laparoscopy in certain circumstances (see p.70).

The operation

Once you have been anaesthetised, you will be placed on your back on the operating table, and your bladder will be catheterised, as described above. A small, usually transverse, incision about 5 to 10 cm (2 to 4 inches) long is made just below the pubic hairline. The surgeon will use forceps to grasp your uterus and pull the fallopian tubes through the incision. Any one of several different methods can be used to remove a segment of each tube. A common method, known as the **Pomeroy**

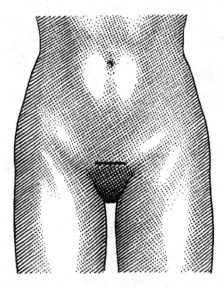

Site of incision for laparotomy for female sterilisation.

method, involves tying an absorbable suture around the base of a loop of the fallopian tube and cutting out a segment of the loop of tube. (This procedure therefore involves both tubal ligation and segmental excision.) The abdominal incision is then closed with dissolvable stitches.

When the suture around the fallopian tube dissolves, the ends of the tube part and the fallopian tube remains occluded.

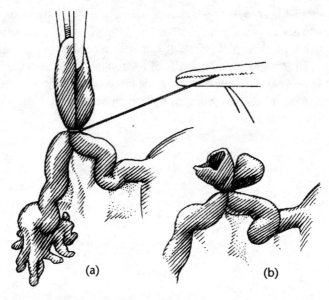

Female sterilisation by ligation and segmental excision. (a) An absorbable suture is tied around a loop of fallopian tube. (b) A segment of the tube is then cut away. When the suture around the fallopian tube dissolves, the ends of the tube part and remain occluded.

When laparotomy is the operation of choice

*   Laparoscopy may be impossible because, for example, a woman has dense pelvic adhesions due to a previous infection or surgery such as repeated caesarean sections.
*   As obesity can make laparoscopic sterilisation more difficult, laparotomy may have to be resorted to for women who are very overweight.
*   Successful laparoscopic operations require a surgeon to have training and practice in specific surgical techniques. Laparotomy may therefore be the operation of choice for some surgeons who lack sufficient experience in laparoscopy

or who do not have access to the necessary equipment.
* If a complication arises during laparoscopic surgery, the operation may have to be completed by laparotomy.
* Laparoscopy is not appropriate for women who are being sterilised at the same time as undergoing another operation, for example a caesarean section or removal of the gall bladder (cholecystectomy). Laparotomy will have been decided on in advance in these cases.
* Although it is no longer common practice to perform sterilisation operations immediately after childbirth, laparotomy is used when they are done at this time. These operations are more likely to be unsuccessful because the fallopian tubes are enlarged following pregnancy. The clips or rings may not be large enough to occlude the entire tube or the rings may remain stretched when the tubes return to their normal size. It is now also recognised that, emotionally, this is not a good time for a woman to undergo sterilisation.

CHAPTER 8

After your operation

AFTER VASECTOMY

You will be able to go home almost immediately after a vasectomy done using a local anaesthetic. However, if you feel faint, you should wait a while until the feeling passes.

It is advisable to attend the clinic for your operation with your partner or a friend who can drive you home afterwards. Although the local anaesthetic will have no effect other than to numb your scrotum, many men do feel a bit unsteady after their operation.

When the anaesthetic wears off, you are likely to have some pain or discomfort in your scrotum, and it is best not to have arranged any activity for at least the rest of that day. Pain-killing tablets such as aspirin or paracetamol, taken regularly, should help to ease any discomfort during the next few hours.

If you have had a general anaesthetic, its effects may last for a day or two (see p.55).

Some GPs like to see their patients a week or so after a vasectomy operation to check that all is well, but others do not think this is necessary. If you are worried about anything, do contact the vasectomy clinic or your GP for advice.

Discomfort and swelling

You will probably feel a bit uncomfortable for the first 48 hours after your operation, and may need to continue taking analgesics for a couple of days.

Most men experience bruising and swelling, which may be severe and which may take several days, or weeks, to clear completely (see p.79). Cubes of ice wrapped in a clean tea-towel or a bag of frozen peas held on the scrotum will help to ease the discomfort. Close-fitting underpants such as Y-fronts will support the scrotum and be more comfortable than loose ones or boxer shorts.

Stitches

The stitches in the small wound or wounds in your scrotum will be dissolvable and therefore do not need to be removed. The gauze placed over the wounds in the clinic can be removed the next morning, and you should wash and dry your genital area carefully and regularly to keep it clean. However, you should avoid soaking the wounds as keeping them dry reduces the risk of infection.

You may have a slight, clear discharge from the wounds for a few days as they heal.

Returning to work

If your job involves heavy lifting, it is probably best to take the following day off work. If not, you can return to work the day after your vasectomy.

Sexual intercourse

It is important to have intercourse regularly after your operation so that the sperm remaining in the vasa deferentia are completely cleared from them. The presence of sperm in the post-operative semen samples (see below) is usually due to infrequent sex in the weeks immediately after surgery; failure of the operation may also be the cause, although this is not common.

Sexual intercourse can be resumed as soon as you feel comfortable. Some form of contraception should be used until you have produced two clear specimens of semen. Your enjoyment of sex should not be affected following your operation, and it may indeed be improved if you have been worried about your partner becoming pregnant.

Semen samples

You will be given written instructions about when and how to obtain the two samples of semen required before you can be considered sterile. You will probably be given two specimen jars before you leave the clinic, with an explanation of where to send these. The first sample is usually required 16 weeks after a vasectomy, and the second 4 weeks after that. You should make sure that you send your samples on the dates indicated, or telephone to warn the appropriate department if you are unable to do so.

You are unlikely to be told of the results of the microscopic examination of your samples until several days after you have despatched the *second*. If both samples are completely free of sperm, you will either receive a letter telling you so or will be told to contact your GP for the results. You can then stop using any other form of contraceptive.

If either of your semen samples still contains sperm, you will be sent another two specimen jars with further dates for posting them. Two consecutive clear samples must be obtained before the vasectomy can be considered to have been successful.

You can fill your specimen jars either by withdrawal during intercourse before ejaculation, or by masturbation into the container itself or into a condom which is then emptied into the container. The condom itself should not be left in the specimen jar.

AFTER TUBAL LIGATION

Effects of the general anaesthetic

You will probably feel drowsy, and possibly nauseated, for a few hours after your operation until the effect of the general anaesthetic wears off. You may also have a sore throat due to the tube which was inserted into your throat to help you breathe while you were anaesthetised. This should improve within a day or two.

Laparoscopy

If your operation is done as day-case surgery, you will be able to go home within a few hours, once you have come round from the anaesthetic and have been seen by a doctor to make sure all is well. At most, you are likely to have to remain in hospital for only one night after your operation. Medical staff will have to be sure that you have recovered sufficiently from the anaesthetic, that there are no apparent complications, and that there will be someone to care for you at home for the next few hours at least.

Discomfort
Some of the gas used to inflate your abdominal cavity during the operation may remain trapped under your diaphragm for a day or two before it is absorbed and expired from your body. This may cause colicky abdominal pain, and possibly referred pain in your shoulder which may be quite severe but which should ease off within a few hours. Your abdomen may feel tender and be swollen for a few days, but if you take things easy for a while, this should soon settle down.

The regular use of painkillers such as aspirin or paracetamol will help to ease any discomfort or pain following your operation.

Stitches
The two small incisions in your abdomen will probably have been closed with stitches which will dissolve within a couple of weeks. However, if these cause irritation or discomfort as the wounds heal, you can make an appointment for the nurse at your GP's surgery to remove them.

Returning to normal activity
You can eat as soon as you want to after your operation, and there are no restrictions on what you eat.

Most women need only three to four days off work following

laparoscopic tubal ligation, during which time they can return gradually to normal activity.

Sexual intercourse can be resumed as soon as it feels comfortable. It is often advised that you continue contraceptive precautions until after your next period. If you wish to stop before this, ask you doctor when it will be safe to do so.

Laparotomy

You may have to spend two or three days in hospital following laparotomy – a more invasive operation than laparoscopy.

Discomfort

As the single incision for laparotomy is larger than the two incisions for laparoscopy, you are likely to have a little more discomfort from your wound after this operation. Regular analgesic tablets will help to control any pain, but do ask a nurse or doctor about pain-killing injections if you feel you need them in the first few post-operative hours.

If you suffer worsening or severe pain in the days after your operation, contact the hospital or your GP so that its cause can be investigated (see Chapter 9).

Stitches

You need to know before you leave hospital whether or not the stitches in your wound(s) are absorbable. If not, they will probably have to be removed five to seven days after your operation. Once you are at home you should make an appointment with the nurse at your GP's surgery for this to be done.

Returning to normal activity

Although you may be fit enough to return to work after a week or so, you should avoid *heavy* lifting for the first six post-operative weeks. Therefore, if your job involves hard physical work, you may need to talk to your GP about taking more time off.

As with a laparoscopic operation, you can resume sexual intercourse as soon as you want to.

Urinary problems

If, as occasionally happens, you are unable to pass urine spontaneously in the first few hours after your operation, a catheter may be inserted to drain the urine from your bladder. This is a painless, although possibly uncomfortable, procedure involving the insertion of a thin tube, coated in anaesthetic, into your urethra. The catheter is unlikely to be required for longer than the first post-operative night.

Following any type of sterilisation operation, you will probably be given a letter for your doctor when you leave the hospital or clinic. You should try to deliver or post it as soon as possible so that your GP is aware of the details of your operation.

CHAPTER 9

Possible complications

Although there are few significant complications associated with either tubal ligation or vasectomy, some problems can arise, as with almost any type of operation. For example, blood clots in the deep veins, normally in the legs (deep vein thrombosis), and clots or air bubbles in the lungs (pulmonary embolism) can occur, although these are very rare after sterilisation operations as the length of time people are immobilised during surgery is so short.

GENERAL COMPLICATIONS

Wound infection

Increased pain or swelling in your wound, or the continued discharge of bloody fluid or of pus, may be a sign that an infection is developing or has developed. Wound infection is rare after laparoscopic sterilisation, but occurs slightly more often following laparotomy. An infected wound will become red, hot to the touch, swollen and tender. You may also have a raised body temperature and feel generally unwell. Infected fluid (pus) may collect in an **abscess** in the wound and, if this occurs, you should seek medical attention. Wound infection may respond to simple cleansing, or antibiotics may be required.

In rare cases of wound infection following laparotomy, some of the stitches may have to be removed from the wound to allow any trapped infected discharge to escape.

Haematoma

A haematoma is a collection of blood which causes a swelling, usually about the size of a grape or larger, which can occur following any type of operation. Haematomas are, however, rare after sterilisation operations. They develop when a blood vessel continues to bleed, or re-opens, following surgery, and are accompanied by pain, a hard swelling, and possibly a reddish purple discoloration of the surrounding skin. Although haematomas are likely to be reabsorbed naturally within three or four weeks, you should seek your doctor's advice if you suspect this complication as it may be necessary for you to have a small operation to close off a vessel if bleeding continues.

Chest infection

Chest infection can occur following the use of a general anaesthetic for any operation, and is more common in heavy smokers. If you start to develop a cold before your operation, it may be better for surgery to be postponed. If you are in any doubt, you should discuss this with the anaesthetist.

FOLLOWING VASECTOMY

Short-term complications

There are several short-term complications which sometimes occur following a vasectomy, but these are rarely serious. Except where their work involves heavy lifting, most men can return to work the day after their operation.

Bruising and swelling
Immediately after surgery, there may be quite severe bruising and swelling of the scrotum, which may remain for two to three

weeks. Swelling and discomfort can be reduced by wearing close-fitting underpants, both day and night, and by the regular use of painkillers. If you do suffer bruising and discomfort, heavy lifting and vigorous sports activity should be avoided for at least a week, i.e. no football, squash or sex. Otherwise, it is perfectly all right to do anything you feel up to.

Persistent, painful swelling or bruising may be due to the collection of blood in a large haematoma (see p.79). If this does occur, you should see your GP or contact the clinic or hospital where your operation was performed as you may need to take antibiotics for a few days to prevent infection until the swelling goes down and the haematoma disperses. Underpants which provide good support will help.

Rarely, it is necessary to drain out infected blood from a haematoma under general anaesthetic. This will require a stay in hospital of a couple of days so that the wound in your scrotum can be re-opened. Small drainage tubes may be left in the re-closed wound for about 48 hours to remove any infected fluid and blood. Once these drains are removed, you will be able to return home, where your wound will have to be dressed regularly for about ten days by a district nurse or at the out-patients' department of a hospital. If the wound has been left open, further admission to hospital may be necessary later for it to be closed again under general anaesthetic.

Wound infection

This is not a very common complication following vasectomy. When it does occur, it may result from infection of a small haematoma (see above) or inflammation of the epididymis.

If the wound continues to be red, swollen and painful, or you develop a temperature, you should seek advice from your doctor so that you can start taking a course of antibiotics as soon as possible.

Sperm granuloma

In the slightly longer term, an epididymis may become tender and possibly swell, forming a lump known as a sperm granuloma. Sperm continue to be produced after vasectomy but, as they are unable to pass through the vas deferens, they are normally simply absorbed by the body. It is thought that granulomas are caused by sperm leaking into the tissues between the cut ends of the vas deferens and triggering a foreign body reaction and inflammation. If the condition persists, it can be treated by the removal of the epididymis under general anaesthetic.

Sperm antibodies

In about 60 to 80 per cent of men who have had vasectomies, the body's immune system reacts to produce antibodies to the sperm which continue to be produced. Although this does not appear to give rise to any symptoms, reversal of the vasectomy may be less likely to be effective.

Long-term complications

There are really no long-term complications following vasectomy, and the operation has no effect on the male hormones or on sexual libido.

At one time there was concern that vasectomy was associated with an increased incidence of heart disease. This suspicion resulted from research done with monkeys fed a very rich and high-fat diet: those monkeys which had had vasectomies were found to be more at risk of developing heart disease. However, the work was not statistically sound, and the theory has since been disproved.

There is inconclusive evidence to suggest a connection between vasectomy and prostate cancer, although none that indicates the operation *causes* this type of cancer. Nor is there evidence of any link with testicular cancer.

Regret
Some men experience regret following a vasectomy, possibly because their circumstances change in ways they could not foresee when they made their decision to be sterilised. Careful thought and counselling from your doctor before your operation should lessen the chances of this occurring.

Scrotal pain
A small minority of men may experience unexplained scrotal pain or discomfort long after their vasectomies, although examination and investigation by a specialist usually fail to reveal any underlying abnormality. Treatment is occasionally necessary to relieve the pain.

FOLLOWING TUBAL LIGATION

There are few serious complications following female sterilisation.

At one time, it was thought that sterilisation caused the menstrual periods to become heavier, but this is now known not to be the case. There is no increased risk of abdominal pain or disturbance of the periods, nor of weight gain, changes in libido, or the need for subsequent gynaecological surgery.

Short-term complications

Urine retention
Very rarely, a woman may have to stay in hospital longer than anticipated following a sterilisation operation because she has difficulty in passing urine. If this occurs, a catheter will have to be passed up the urethra to drain the urine from the bladder.

You will then have to stay in hospital at least overnight until the catheter can be removed and you are able to pass urine spontaneously.

Pain

If you do have undue pain after your operation, you may be kept in hospital a little longer so that you can be given adequate pain-relieving drugs and be observed to make sure the laparoscope has not damaged your bowel or caused excessive bleeding (see below).

Effects of the anaesthetic

You may suffer from nausea or vomiting and feel generally poorly for a day or two after your operation until the effects of the general anaesthetic wear off. Most women need to stay off work for at least two to three days.

You may have a sore throat due to the 'dry' anaesthetic gases used or to the tube which was passed down your throat during your operation. This should improve within a couple of days.

Accidental damage

Even operations performed by the most experienced surgeons can occasionally result in accidental damage to a large blood vessel or organ such as the bladder or small or large bowel. The laparoscope may tear through a fallopian tube, possibly causing bleeding into the abdomen or broad ligament. Such accidents are rare, but when they do occur laparotomy is necessary to repair the damage.

Long-term complications

Regret

Women, like men, can experience regret after sterilisation. The decision to undergo this operation should never be made at a time of emotional or other upset, for example in an attempt to save a rocky marriage. This is one reason why sterilisation is now rarely thought appropriate immediately after childbirth or the stillbirth of a child. Other forms of contraception should always be considered carefully first, and an effort should be made to try to imagine circumstances in which your desire to have no more children could change (see Chapter 3).

Pregnancy

Pregnancy is uncommon after tubal ligation, but when it does occur there is an increased risk of it being ectopic (see p.25).

It is most likely that your post-operative recovery will be straightforward and uneventful. However, do contact your GP, the hospital ward or clinic, or your consultant if you are at all concerned about anything that occurs.

CHAPTER 10

Private care

There are various reasons why people choose to have their operations done privately. They may have private health insurance,
or be covered by a private health scheme run by the company
for which they work, or they may be able to pay for private care
themselves. Whatever your reason, you will not find that the
standard of medical care you receive in a private hospital is any
different from that available on the National Health Service
(NHS). However, you may prefer the privacy of a private hospital; or you may find the much-reduced waiting time to see a consultant, and the opportunity to enter hospital for your operation
at the time of your choice are more convenient for you. If you
have an operation in an NHS hospital, you may rarely see the
consultant, being examined and treated by different doctors in
the consultant's firm. At a private hospital, you will receive personal care from the consultant throughout your stay. The facilities at a private hospital are likely to be more like those of a
good hotel, and will certainly include a private bathroom.

The information given in other chapters in this book is equally
relevant whichever system you choose. This chapter deals with
those aspects of private health care which differ from those of
the NHS.

PRIVATE HEALTH INSURANCE

Most private health insurance schemes do *not* cover sterilisation
operations, so you will need to check your policy carefully to
find out if yours does. If the company you work for has a private

health insurance scheme, your Company Secretary will be able to give you the relevant details.

If you have your own private health insurance and it is not clear from the literature you already have whether sterilisation is included, the insurance company will be able to tell you exactly what is covered by your particular policy.

There are different levels of health insurance, and you need to make sure you know precisely which costs are covered by your policy. Most private hospitals have an administration officer who will check this for you if you are in any doubt. The staff at the hospital are likely to be very helpful and will try to sort out any problems and queries you have. But do read your policy carefully, and any information sent to you by the hospital, as unexpected charges, such as consultants' fees that you thought were covered, could add up to quite a lot of money.

With some types of private health insurance, operations can only be undertaken if a GP fills in a form stating that surgery is necessary and cannot be done in an NHS hospital within a certain time period due to long waiting lists.

FIXED PRICE CARE

You may be in the position of being able to pay to have your operation done privately. The Bookings Manager at a private hospital will be able to give you an idea of the cost involved. At current prices, laparoscopic sterilisation costs around £1000, and vasectomy under local anaesthetic around £220. However, these are only approximate prices, and the actual costs may vary.

Some private hospitals run a service known as Fixed Price Care: a price can be quoted to you before you enter hospital which covers your operation and a variety of other hospitalisation costs. You should always ask to have the quotation in writing *before* you enter hospital, with a written note of everything it covers. At some hospitals, the fixed price will include accommodation, nursing, meals, drugs, dressings, operating theatre fees, X-rays etc.; at others only some of these costs are covered. Once you have a quotation, you should not have to worry about any hidden costs which you had not accounted for. However, the price quoted to you by the hospital may not include the fees of the consultant surgeon or consultant anaesthetist, and you may have to ask your consultant for a note of these.

With Fixed Price Care, all the hospitalisation costs included by that particular hospital are covered should you need to stay longer than expected in hospital (usually up to a maximum of 28 days) as a direct result of complications arising from your operation. In other words, if you develop some problem while in hospital that is unrelated to the sterilisation operation itself, the price you have been quoted will not cover treatment to deal with this. If, on the other hand, a complication arises as a direct result of the operation, and your consultant decides to keep you in hospital for longer than originally planned, all the costs which arise from your stay and are included in the hospital's fixed price (again, with the possible exception of consultants' fees) will be covered. At some hospitals, the quoted price will also cover your treatment should you have to be re-admitted due to a complication related to your original operation and arising within a limited period of time after your original discharge.

The only extra charges that you will have to pay to the hospital will probably include those for telephone calls, any alcohol if you have this with your meals, food provided for your visitors, personal laundry done by the hospital, hairdressing, and for any similar items such as you would have to pay for in a hotel. It is usually possible for a visitor to eat meals with you in your room, and for tea and snacks to be ordered for visitors during the day. (You will also have to pay these extra charges before you leave the hospital if you are being treated under private health insurance.)

It is important therefore that you ask in advance for *written* confirmation of the price you will have to pay for your stay in hospital and what is included in the quotation. If the hospital does not have a Fixed Price Care or similar system, make sure that all possible costs are listed.

ARRANGING THE OPERATION

Although the medical treatment you receive in a private hospital will be similar to that available at any NHS hospital, there are some basic differences between the two systems.

As with the NHS, you will have to be referred to see a consultant privately by your GP. Most GPs have contacts with particular consultants (and private hospitals) to whom they tend to refer patients. If there is a private hospital you particularly want to go to, or a consultant you have some reason to prefer, you can ask your GP to make an appointment for you.

After your visit to your GP, you are unlikely to have to wait longer than a week or two before you see the consultant at an out-patient appointment. Your appointment may be at the private hospital where your operation is to be carried out, at an NHS hospital which has private wards, or at the consultant's private consulting rooms. Once the decision has been made to go ahead with surgery, you will probably be able to enter hospital at your convenience within another week or two.

You will receive confirmation of the date of your operation from the Bookings Manager of the hospital you are to attend. You will also probably be sent leaflets and any further relevant details of how to prepare for your admission to hospital. Do read these carefully, as knowing how your particular hospital organises things will help you to be prepared when you arrive for your operation. You will also be sent a pre-admission form to fill in and take with you when you are admitted.

If your operation is being paid for by insurance, you will be asked to take a completed insurance form with you when you are admitted to hospital. You should have been given some of these forms when you first took out your policy, but your insurance company will be able to supply the correct form if you have any problems. If you are covered by company insurance, the form will probably be filled in and given to you by your Company Secretary.

ADMISSION TO HOSPITAL

When you arrive at the hospital, the receptionist will contact the admissions department, and a ward receptionist will come to collect you. If you are paying for your stay in hospital yourself, you will probably be asked to pay your bill in advance at this stage if you have not already done so. Otherwise, you will be asked for your completed insurance form. The ward receptionist will take you to your room – probably a single or double room – and show you the facilities available there. You are likely to have a private bathroom, a television, and a telephone by your bed. The ward receptionist will explain hospital procedures to you, and will leave you to settle in.

A member of the nursing staff will then come to make a note of your medical details. If you have been treated in an NHS hospital before, the main difference you are likely to notice is that this time there is much less waiting for all the routine hospital procedures to be dealt with. The nurse to patient ratio is higher in private hospitals and so someone is usually available to deal with the pre-operative procedures quite quickly.

Your consultant will take charge of your medical care throughout your stay, will visit you before the operation, perform the operation (with the assistance of the anaesthetist and the operating staff), and visit you again when you are back in your own room. Trainees – whether doctors or nurses – do not work in private hospitals. The consultants are responsible for their own patients and supervise their care themselves. Most private hospitals now have resident medical officers – fully qualified, regis-tered doctors who are available 24 hours a day to deal with any emergencies which may arise.

PREPARING FOR YOUR OPERATION

If you are having a general anaesthetic, a porter and nurse will take you from your room to the anaesthetic room when the time for your operation approaches. In many private hospitals, you will not be moved from your bed onto a trolley until you have been anaesthetised; the bed itself will be wheeled from your room. Similarly, you will be transferred back from the trolley to your own bed in the recovery room while you are still asleep. You therefore go to sleep and wake up in your own hospital bed.

If you are having a local anaesthetic, you will be able to walk to the operating room.

Your operation will be performed in the same way as described in Chapters 6 and 7. When you are fully awake, you will be taken back to your room to rest.

DISCHARGE FROM HOSPITAL

When you are ready to be discharged from hospital, the ward receptionist will ask you to pay any outstanding charges not covered by the hospitalisation charge. You will be given any medical items you may need from the hospital pharmacy.

DIFFERENCES AND SIMILARITIES

The main aim of the staff of any private hospital is the same as that in an NHS hospital – to make your stay as pleasant and as comfortable as possible. Because the staffing ratio is higher in private hospitals, more emphasis can be placed on privacy and comfort.

The consultant surgeons and anaesthetists almost always work in an NHS hospital as well as in a private hospital, so you will receive the same expertise and skill under both systems. However, in an NHS hospital you may not actually be operated on by the consultant surgeon who heads the surgical team, and, indeed, you may not see the consultant at all during your stay.

Private hospitals arrange their operating lists differently from NHS hospitals. The latter have 'sessional bookings' for their operating theatres. This means a particular day is set aside at regular intervals for a specialist in one type of surgery to perform operations. In private hospitals, the consultants can book the use of an operating theatre (and the assistance of the staff who work in it) on any day, at any time that suits them. Therefore, your operation can take place privately with minimum delay, and at a time that is convenient to you and your consultant. The shorter waiting lists for sterilisation operations are perhaps the main advantage of private care in this instance.

It is also possible, even if you are already on an NHS waiting list, to tell your GP or consultant at any time that you would like to change to private care. If the consultant you have already seen under the NHS does not have a private practice, you can ask to be put in touch with one who *can* see you privately.

SUMMARY

There are several reasons why, if they can, some people choose to have their operations done privately, either paid for by private health insurance or from their own pockets. Some find it much more convenient to be able to have a say in when their operation is to take place. The NHS, under which the majority of people are treated, naturally has longer waiting lists. If time is an important factor for you, you may be happy to pay to have your operation done at a time that you find convenient.

Some people simply prefer the smaller, more intimate setting they are likely to find in a private hospital. Private hospitals rarely deal with accidents and emergency treatment; the operations carried out in them are normally planned, at least a day or two in advance. Therefore, they do not have the bustle of an NHS hospital which has to deal with emergency admissions as well as the routine admissions for non-emergency operations.

Questions and answers

1.   *I am 26 and my husband is 28. We have two children and are both sure that we do not want any more. I would like to be sterilised as I do not always remember to take the contraceptive pill. Is my doctor likely to agree to my request?*

Different doctors may have different opinions on whether you are too young to be considering sterilisation. If your GP has known you for some time, and feels that you and your husband will have thought carefully about your decision, he or she may be happy to refer you to a consultant. You are unlikely to be *refused* the operation – by either your GP or consultant – but may be advised to think again because of your relatively young ages. Do listen to any advice you are offered: doctors quite often come across people who regret having been sterilised. It may be suggested that you try a contraceptive implant or injections as these are reversible forms of contraception which would deal with the problem of forgetting to take your pill. If you are determined to be sterilised, perseverance is likely to pay off in the end.

2.   *I am 33, married, with no children. My husband and I have decided that we do not want a family, and I would like to be sterilised. However, my GP has advised me against this and she did not seem to be prepared to refer me to a consultant. What can I do?*

If you are absolutely sure that sterilisation is the right answer for you, your GP should refer you to a consultant if requested to do so. She may have good reasons for feeling your decision is inappropriate, which she should have explained to you. However, the decision is ultimately yours. Your doctor can only really advise you from her own professional experience. It may be worth talking to a doctor at a family planning clinic who would also be able to refer you to a consultant.

3. *My wife wants me to be sterilised as we have three children and do not want any more. However, I do not really want to have a vasectomy, although I understand her point that it is a simpler operation for me. Are there any equally satisfactory alternatives?*

Apart from condoms, vasectomy is the only feasible alternative form of contraception currently available for men in the UK. It is a relatively minor operation and, as it involves only a local anaesthetic, does not carry any of the risks associated with the general anaesthesia usually necessary for female sterilisation. However, if your concerns relate to the finality of the operation as a form of contraception, it would be worth discussing them further with your GP or a doctor at a family planning clinic and with your wife, on whom any failure of contraception will have a more direct effect. Ultimately, the decision to have any operation must be made by the person who is having it done.

4. *I had a tubal ligation about five years ago, but have since divorced and remarried and would now like to have another child. Is a reversal of the operation possible?*

When choosing sterilisation as a form of contraception, people are always told that they should view it as an irreversible procedure. Surgery to reverse tubal ligation is much more complicated than the tubal ligation itself and requires a longer time under general anaesthetic. Your GP may be able to refer you to a surgeon with experience in this type of surgery, but even if the surgeon agrees to attempt reversal, its success will depend in part on the condition of the remains of your fallopian tubes.

There must be enough healthy tube left for the severed ends to be rejoined, and this will only be apparent once an operation has begun. However, even after an apparently successful operation, fertility may not be restored. Your GP or a doctor at a family planning clinic should be able to advise you, and can also tell you whether or not this operation is available under the NHS in your area.

5. *I am 42 and have been considering sterilisation for a couple of years. However, a friend of mine who recently had a hysterectomy suggested that I ask my GP about this as it would also save me any possible troubles later. Is my doctor likely to agree to this?*

If there is no medical reason why you require a hysterectomy, such as heavy or irregular periods which are making your life difficult, no doctor is likely to agree to your undergoing this major form of surgery simply as a method of contraception. Sterilisation is a far more appropriate option for you.

6. *I have very heavy periods which are often accompanied by quite severe pains. Would a sterilisation operation cure these menstrual problems?*

Sterilisation is extremely unlikely to have any effect on your periods, except possibly in the very short term. A hysterectomy may be an option, and you should discuss this possibility with your GP. Removal of the womb would, of course, also render you sterile.

7. *I am 44 and am waiting to have a sterilisation operation. However, I am becoming increasingly worried about having a general anaesthetic, which I understand is the normal type of anaesthesia for tubal ligation. Is there an alternative?*

The majority of female sterilisation operations are done using a general anaesthetic, but it is sometimes possible to have local anaesthesia instead. You should explain your worries to your consultant, and ask about any alternatives available. There are a couple of clinics at which female sterilisations are routinely done using local anaesthesia (the Elliot Smith Clinic in the Churchill Hospital, Oxford, and the Margaret Pike Clinic in London), and if you are able to pay to have your operation, it may be worth asking for details from one of these.

8. My wife and I are considering sterilisation (we are both in our late forties). Is there any reason why it is better for one of us to have an operation rather than the other?

A vasectomy is a less invasive operation than tubal ligation and avoids any of the risks inherent in the use of general anaesthesia. However, the reverse side of the coin is that your wife is naturally approaching the end of her reproductive life and would be less likely to want, or be able to have, any more children should your marriage ever break down. You, on the other hand, will probably continue to be fertile for some years to come. If you are both sure that your marriage is secure, or that you yourself would not want more children should anything happen to your wife, then, practically, it may be better for you to have a vasectomy.

9. I am pregnant and about to have my third child. I asked my GP about being sterilised while I am in hospital giving birth, but she advised me against this. Why?

Experience has shown that women are more likely to regret being sterilised when the operation is done at a time of emotional upset, including immediately after childbirth. It is also a time when you will want, if possible, to be awake and with your baby. A sterilisation done at this time may leave you feeling groggy for a day or so, and possibly sore and uncomfortable.

10. *I am due to have my baby by caesarean section, and wonder if I could be sterilised at the same time?*

You should ask your consultant or GP about this in good time, and be absolutely sure that it is what you want to do. It may be possible for sterilisation to be carried out immediately after the birth of your baby, and this is an exception to the normally applied rule of avoiding sterilisation at the time of childbirth as an operation is being performed anyway. However, there is a higher failure rate when sterilisation is done immediately following childbirth (both natural and by caesarean section) as the fallopian tubes enlarge during pregnancy, and the rings placed over them may become loose when the tubes shrink back to their normal size.

11. *I recently had a sterilisation operation which involved quite a large wound being made in my lower abdomen. Although it seemed all right when I was in hospital, it has now become hard and sore and is very red. Is this normal, and if not, what should I do about it?*

It is possible that you have an infection in the wound and you should therefore seek medical advice from your GP so that it can be checked and cleaned. You may need to have a course of antibiotics, and if pus from the wound collects in an abscess, this will also need attention. Wound infections are not uncommon, and although there is unlikely to be any real cause for concern, they should always be looked at by a doctor as soon as possible.

12. *An appointment has been made for me to have a sterilisation operation during a time when my husband will be away. As I have waited several months for this operation, I do not want to have to postpone it. Will I be able to come home immediately afterwards and be able to look after our two children alone?*

If your operation is to be done laparoscopically, you will probably be able to return home within a few hours, once you have recovered from the anaesthetic. However, you will need a responsible adult to care for you, at least overnight, as the effects of the anaesthetic take a while to wear off. You really should arrange for someone to be there when you get home from hospital and to help you care for your children, at least until the following day. You should also bear in mind that if a minor complication arises during or after your operation, you may have to stay a little longer in hospital and cannot therefore be sure to be home at a specific time.

13.   My sterilisation operation has been cancelled twice. My consultant says that there is nothing he can do about this and that he will fit me in again as soon as he can. Is there anything I can do to speed things up?

It may be worth contacting your District Health Authority to explain the situation and the difficulties you have had, although it is likely that your consultant will be aware of the distress the cancellations have caused you and will make every effort to fit your operation in to his schedule as soon as possible. Sterilisation is not an urgent operation, and may well be the one that is cancelled if an emergency arises. You have been unlucky to have it postponed twice, but there is probably nothing you can do except try to be patient, and perhaps write to the consultant to remind him that you are still waiting.

14.   An appointment has been made for me to see a male consultant about a tubal ligation. Is it possible for me to ask to see a woman instead?

You should certainly tell your GP that you would prefer to see a woman, and every effort should be made to meet this request, although the majority of gynaecologists are still men and it may simply not be possible to do so. You may have to go to a hospital outside your immediate area, if this can be arranged.

15. How long will I have to remain in hospital following a laparotomy for sterilisation?

Laparotomy is a more invasive operation than laparoscopic ster-ilisation, and you may have to remain in hospital for two or three nights after it. The wound made in your abdomen will be larger than those made for laparoscopy, and you may need more pain relief for a day or two post-operatively. There is also more chance of minor post-operative complications, such as urine retention or wound infection, and you will be kept under medical super-vision until medical staff are happy that all seems to be well.

16. I am due to have a vasectomy next month, for which I have been waiting some time. However, I am now not sure I want to have the oper-ation, but am embarrassed to tell my doctor as I feel I have already been a bit of a nuisance. Should I just go ahead, and hope that it can be reversed if I ever change my mind?

No! Sterilisation should always be considered to be irreversible, and should never be undergone by anyone who is not com-pletely sure that they have made the right decision. Your doctor should certainly not feel you are being a nuisance, and should be sympathetic to your anxiety. You may want to discuss things again with your GP or with a doctor at a family planning clinic before you ask for your operation to be cancelled. Only you can make this decision, and embarrassment at 'feeling a nuisance' should not be a factor under any circumstances.

17. I had a vasectomy about three years ago, but my wife has now become pregnant. She says that the baby is mine, and I have no reason to doubt her, except that I thought is was not possible for me to father a child as I no longer produce any sperm.

Vasectomy has no effect on the production of sperm. It simply involves severing of the vasa deferentia so that the sperm which continue to be produced in the testes cannot escape from them and are reabsorbed by the body. It is possible for a structure other than the vas deferens to be cut during a vasectomy operation, although this very rarely occurs when surgery is performed by experienced surgeons. It is also possible for the two cut ends of a vas deferens to rejoin spontaneously some time after surgery, although again this is not common. There is, therefore, a chance that your vasectomy may have failed, and you should discuss this with your GP, who will probably refer you to a consultant for investigation. Apart from the need to reassure yourself and to remove any doubts about your wife, if your vasectomy has failed, it is necessary for steps to be taken to ensure that the failure is corrected and cannot happen again.

Normally in cases like yours results of semen tests show a very small number of sperm present, but even a negative test does not preclude the possibility that there may have been sperm in your semen at some point. If the results of tests are inconclusive, you and your wife may want to consider DNA testing of the baby, once born.

18.   Will *a vasectomy reduce my enjoyment of sex*?

A vasectomy should have no effect on your enjoyment of sex, except possibly to improve it if you have been worried about your partner becoming pregnant. You will continue to ejaculate as normal and, once you have recovered from the operation, you should not notice any difference. Vasectomy has no effect on the production of male hormones; it simply prevents release of sperm into the semen.

Case histories

The case histories which follow are not intended to make any specific point. They have been chosen at random as examples of the experiences of different men and women, and are included simply to illustrate the reality of having a sterilisation operation for these people.

CASE 1

Karen is 44, and has three sons aged 21, 24 and 26. Soon after the birth of her youngest child, she discussed sterilisation with her GP, but he felt that she was too young to consider this form of contraception. She therefore began to take a contraceptive pill, and continued to do so for about 10 years. As Karen was a smoker, she then stopped taking the pill and had a coil inserted. Some years later, when her periods became heavy and painful, her GP suggested the coil be removed in case it was the cause of her problems, and he arranged for her to see a consultant at a local hospital.

The consultant agreed that it might be best to remove the coil and Karen decided to be sterilised at the same time. Her husband was not prepared to consider a vasectomy.

The coil was removed, tubal ligation was carried out, and a dilatation and curettage (D & C) operation was done to investigate any other possible cause of Karen's menstrual problems. She was not told the result of the D & C, and assumed that all was well.

After her sterilisation operation, Karen found that not having to worry about becoming pregnant made her feel more relaxed about sexual intercourse. For about a year, her menstrual problems also seemed to have been resolved. However, her periods gradually became heavier, more frequent and painful until, at the age of 44, following discussions with her GP and consultant, she had a hysterectomy.

CASE 2

Sarah is 34, and has three children, aged 5, 9 and 11. A couple of years after the birth of her youngest child, she had an operation to repair her bladder, and was advised not to have any more children. She used a contraceptive pill until her last pregnancy, after which she changed to using a coil. When her periods became heavy and painful, she thought her problems might be due to the coil, and she therefore discussed with her GP the possibility of sterilisation. Her husband was unwilling to consider having a vasectomy. Sarah was not offered any counselling before her operation, but as she had thought carefully about sterilisation, she was happy to go ahead without further discussion. An appointment was made for her to see a consultant a couple of months later. Two months after this, she was admitted to her local hospital at 7.30 in the morning to have day-case surgery for the removal of her coil and for tubal ligation.

When Sarah came round after the operation, she felt quite sick, but the feeling passed after a couple of hours, and she dozed for the rest of the day, leaving hospital at 6 p.m. When she got home, she had something to eat and went to bed. The next morning she awoke feeling fine, and was able to go out. She returned to work the following day.

Sarah did not need painkillers at all after her operation. Her stomach remained swollen for about a week, and tender for a few days longer, although it was not generally painful. She was able to resume sexual intercourse a couple of days after her operation, and her husband used condoms until she had had her next period. A couple of months after her sterilisation operation, the two small scars below Sarah's umbilicus and just above her pubic hairline were barely visible. She is very pleased that she decided to be sterilised.

CASE 3

Elizabeth is 33, with three sons, aged 7, 5 and 2. She decided she would like to be sterilised when her youngest child was about 18 months old. She and her husband (aged 38) felt that their financial situation precluded them having more children and, as her husband is very opposed to abortion, Elizabeth did not like the prospect of possibly having to make a decision alone should she become pregnant again. She was sure that she did not want any more children, and would not do so even if her marriage were to break down and she were to marry again. Elizabeth's husband would not consider a vasectomy, and he was ambivalent about whether he would want more children in other circumstances.

Elizabeth went to talk to her GP, who referred her to a consultant. When she saw the consultant about eight weeks later, an appointment was made for her to have a laparoscopic sterilisation operation. However, the consultant explained that Elizabeth's heavy periods might become heavier when she stopped taking the pill, and suggested that she do so immediately and see what happened during the four months before her operation was scheduled. However, Elizabeth's menstrual bleeding became only slightly heavier, and she did not have any period-related pains.

She was therefore admitted to hospital as planned, arriving at 10.30 in the morning and leaving again at 7 p.m. When she awoke in the recovery room after the operation, she was lying on her side and had pain in her shoulder caused by the gas which had been used to inflate her abdomen. She was given a pain-killing tablet, the only one she had to take throughout her recovery. She had no pain from the small wounds and felt completely recovered within a couple of days, with only slight discomfort and a bloated feeling caused by the residual gas. Her wounds healed quickly, leaving inconspicuous scars, and she was very pleased with the way things had gone.

CASE 4

Rebecca is 25 years old, and has two sons, aged 7 and 5. After her second child was born she was quite sure she did not want any more children. She did ask her GP about the possibility of being sterilised, but he advised her against it because of her age, and she continued taking a contraceptive pill. However, when her younger child was 4 years old, Rebecca was distressed to discover that she was pregnant again, but about eight weeks into the pregnancy she suffered a spontaneous abortion. After this experience, Rebecca's GP agreed to refer her to a consultant to discuss sterilisation, and an appointment was made for some six months later.

The consultant talked to Rebecca about alternative forms of contraception, but she was adamant that she wanted to be sterilised. Although her husband was prepared to have a vasectomy, Rebecca felt that if their marriage should ever break down, it was possible that he would want more children. The consultant suggested that she return three months later, having thought about what they had discussed and having talked it through with her husband. She was admitted to hospital for tubal ligation as a day case about a month after this.

Rebecca was very uncomfortable for three days after her operation, and found it difficult to walk about, and impossible to bend over. She had a small wound in her navel, and another just above her pubic hairline, both of which had been stitched with absorbable stitches. She was told not to get the wounds wet for at least three days as water would dissolve the glue-like substance which had been used to help hold the wound edges together. She had a bath three days after her operation, but shortly afterwards the wound in her navel was pulled open by her jeans, and began to bleed and leak fluid. The nurse at her GP's surgery cleaned the wound and put small adhesive strips over it to hold the edges together. However, these also became unstuck and had to be replaced.

Rebecca found sexual intercourse painful and suffered cramp-like pains after her operation, also finding it difficult and painful to urinate. Her GP gave her antibiotics but these did not improve the situation; a sample of her urine showed no sign of infection. The pains continued for four weeks, throughout which time Rebecca took painkillers regularly, but all her symptoms improved after her first proper period. Since then, her enjoyment of sex has increased.

CASE 5

Harry is 31. His wife is 30 and has two children, aged 11 and 9, from a previous marriage. They also have two children of their own, aged 3 years and 5 months. After the first of their own children was born, they started to think about the possibility of sterilisation. Harry's wife has had a deep vein thrombosis and is therefore unable to take oral contraceptives, so Harry used condoms. When his wife was pregnant with their second child, Harry talked to his doctor about a vasectomy. The births of their children had not been easy for his wife, and he did not want her to undergo sterilisation.

Harry received an appointment for a vasectomy at an evening clinic at a local hospital about ten months after seeing his GP. During the operation, the injection of local anaesthetic into the scrotum was slightly painful, but no more so than other types of injection Harry has had. The operation lasted about 20 minutes, during which time he experienced only a tugging sensation. The next day, he found movement quite painful, but only needed to take painkillers regularly for about 24 hours. Harry is self-employed and was able to take a couple of days off work, staying at home to rest and catch up with his paperwork.

The bruising and swelling of his scrotum were more extensive than he had expected, and a couple of days after his vasectomy he began to have intermittent severe abdominal pains. His GP examined him a few days later and gave him some antibiotics in case the pains were due to an infection. The abdominal pains and swelling made sexual intercourse impossible, but finally cleared up after about ten days.

The jokes made by Harry's friends and colleagues began to tail off after a few weeks, and the whole experience had been far less traumatic than he had anticipated. He and his wife feel that their relationship has improved as a result of his operation.

CASE 6

Paul is 40, his wife is 41, and they have three children. Although he had considered having a vasectomy, it was not until after the unplanned birth of their third child that he made an appointment to see a doctor at a family planning clinic. The condoms he had been using had not proved to be a foolproof method of contraception. Paul was given quite comprehensive counselling, although he had really already made up his mind. An appointment was made for him to have a vasectomy at the family planning clinic. The operation went smoothly and his anxiety about the pain of an injection in the scrotum proved to be unfounded.

Paul's vasectomy was done on a Friday, and he was completely pain free and able to return to work by the Monday. However, about a week after his operation, he began to experience considerable pain and tenderness in his scrotum, which he at first assumed to be a natural result of the surgery. When the tenderness became unbearable, he returned to the family planning clinic for advice. His GP gave him some antibiotics, which for a while seemed to work, but a couple of months later the pain returned. A course of different antibiotics finally resolved the problem. Had he been aware of the possibility of post-operative infection developing, Paul would have sought medical advice as soon as the pain began.

Once the infection had cleared up, Paul was very pleased with the results of his operation, and would recommend it to others.

CASE 7

At the age of 30, Owen was married for the second time and was the father of a child from each marriage. His wife was taking a contraceptive pill, and when they decided they did not want another child, Owen had a vasectomy. However, his second marriage later broke down, and he eventually found a new partner, 17 years younger than himself, who wanted to have at least one child of her own. Owen's inability to have children put a strain on their relationship and, at the age of 45, he went to see a consultant to discuss the possibility of a reversal of his vasectomy. He was told that reversal would have a 50/50 chance of success, and he decided to go ahead. The operation was done privately, with minimum delay, and he stayed overnight in hospital after it. He recovered quickly from the general anaesthetic and suffered very little post-operative pain.

The semen sample Owen supplied some weeks after his operation showed his sperm count to be low, and many of the sperm to be non-viable. Although he was told that he had just over a 1 per cent chance of fathering a child, his partner conceived within four months of the operation. Since the birth of their child, she has been taking a contraceptive pill.

CASE 8

Kevin had a vasectomy at the age of 28, when he and his wife had two children. Their relationship seemed stable, and their economic situation at the time was such that their standard of living could only be maintained if they both worked. Neither Kevin nor his wife saw the pill as a suitable long-term contraceptive option.

About three years after his vasectomy, Kevin's marriage broke down, and at the age of 32 he met someone else. They were married four years later. His new wife is eight years younger than Kevin and had not had any children. Her decision to marry Kevin knowing she was unlikely ever to have any was therefore a hard one to make. They did discuss the possibility of a reversal operation before they were married, and afterwards Kevin saw a consultant privately to find out about it. The consultant said that reversal was possible but that its chances of success were low – about 30 per cent. The operation was done under the NHS a couple of months later.

When Kevin supplied his semen sample he was told that the reversal had failed and that his semen did not contain sperm. The doctor he saw at the hospital said that nothing further could be done. Kevin was insistent and finally the doctor gave him the name of a consultant with experience of similar problems. When Kevin saw this consultant privately he was told that there should be no problem in attempting another reversal and that it could be done under the NHS. However, he decided to have it done privately to ensure that the consultant himself would do the operation, and it was carried out within a few weeks.

Kevin's first semen sample some three months later showed the presence of sperm, although they were of low motility. A second sample revealed a good sperm count with increased motility.

Kevin's wife conceived within six months of his second reversal operation, and they now have a 6-year-old and a 6-month-old child. At the age of 44, Kevin underwent a second vasectomy operation.

Medical terms

Abdomen/Abdominal cavity The body cavity between the diaphragm and the floor of the pelvis which contains the organs of digestion – the stomach and intestines.

Abscess A pus-filled cavity which has developed as a result of the disintegration of tissue.

Absorbable sutures/stitches Sutures which are made of a material which is able to dissolve in the tissues, such as catgut or the synthetic fibre Vicryl. Absorbable sutures do not need to be removed.

Adhesion The joining together of parts of the body which are normally separate.

Allergy An over-sensitivity to a particular substance which causes the body to react against it. An **allergic reaction** may be mild, such as an itchy rash, or it may be more severe, involving fainting, vomiting or loss of consciousness. Your doctor should be told about any allergies you have so that they can be added to your medical records.

Anaesthetic A drug which causes loss of sensation in part of the body and/or loss of consciousness.

Analgesic A drug which blocks sensations of pain; a pain-killer.

Antibiotic A substance which kills or prevents the reproduction of bacteria.

Antibody A protein produced by the body in response to the presence of cells which are perceived as 'foreign' to it (antigens). Antibodies form an important part of the body's defence mechanism against illness and disease.

Anti-embolism stockings/Compression stockings/Thrombo-embolic deterrent stockings (TEDS) Stockings worn by patients during and after an operation to help prevent blood clots forming in the deep veins of the legs. The stockings work by assisting the circulation of the blood within the veins of the legs.

Anti-emetic A drug which helps to stop you vomiting or feeling sick.

Barrier methods of contraception Various contraceptive methods which involve the use of a physical barrier to prevent contact between sperm and ova, for example condoms and caps.

Blood clot A solidified mass of blood.

Broad ligament A strand of membrane attached to either side of the uterus and to the ovaries which connects them to the abdominal wall and helps to hold them in place within the abdominal cavity.

Bruise The discoloration caused by blood accumulating in the tissues under the skin in the area of an injury.

Caesarean section Delivery of a fetus through an incision made in the mother's abdominal wall and in the wall of her uterus.

Cannula A very fine tube or needle which is inserted into a vein, usually in the back of the hand. Cannulas are used to introduce or remove fluids from the body, and to administer drugs such as anaesthetics. They are usually made of flexible plastic, but can be glass or metal. A common variety is the butterfly cannula.

Cap A contraceptive device which can be inserted by a woman into her vagina before sexual intercourse and which covers the cervix, thus preventing sperm entering the uterus and fertilising an ovum.

Catheter A thin tube used to withdraw or introduce fluid into the body. Bladder catheters are inserted through the urethra into the bladder to drain the urine from it.

Cervical smear test   The removal of a small sample of cells from the cervix of the uterus for examination under a microscope. The cells are scraped from the cervix using a specially shaped wooden spatula. The test is done to detect early precancerous cell changes which identify women at high risk of developing cervical cancer.

Cervix   The lower part of the uterus where it protrudes into the vagina.

Coil   A plastic contraceptive device, with or without a copper wire coiled around the stem, which is inserted into the uterine cavity.

Complication   A condition which occurs as a result of another disease or treatment, e.g. infection of a wound following surgery.

Condom   Most commonly, a latex sheath which can be fitted over the erect penis before sexual intercourse to collect ejaculated semen and prevent the sperm contained in it from entering the woman's vagina. Condoms are also available for use by women: they are polyurethane sheaths which can be inserted into the vagina.

Consent form   A form which patients must sign before surgery to confirm that their treatment has been explained to them, that they understand what is to take place and have given their permission for the operation and anaesthesia.

Contraception   Any method of preventing pregnancy.

Contraceptive implant   A small hormone-containing device which can be placed under the skin through a small incision, usually in the arm. The hormone is slowly released and prevents conception occurring. The most commonly used implant in the UK is **Norplant**, which remains effective for about five years.

Contraceptive injection   An intramuscular injection of contraceptive hormone which is effective in preventing conception for 8 (**Noristerat**) or 12 (**Depo-provera**) weeks.

Contraceptive sponge   A foam sponge impregnated with a

spermicide which can be inserted by a woman into her vagina before sexual intercourse. The sponge acts both as a physical barrier to the passage of sperm and to absorb some of the semen entering the vagina.

Corpus (of uterus)   The body of the uterus.

Corpus luteum   The yellow body which remains after an ovarian follicle has ruptured and released it ovum. It produces the hormone progesterone.

Culdotomy   A surgical procedure in which an incision is made in the top of the vagina through which the fallopian tubes can be pulled to be cut away. This form of sterilisation is now rarely performed.

Cystitis   Inflammation of the bladder due to injury or infection.

Day-case surgery   Any operation carried out on a patient who is in hospital for one day only, with no overnight stay.

Deep vein thrombosis   A blood clot in the deep veins of the body, normally in the legs or pelvis.

Depo-provera   A contraceptive injection, the effects of which last for about 12 weeks.

Diaphragm   A small rubber disc which can be inserted by a woman into her vagina before sexual intercourse to form a physical barrier to the passage of sperm into the uterus. Diaphragms should always be used with a spermicide.

Diathermy   The process by which heat is applied to the tissues to stop bleeding during an operation. The heat is usually provided by a high-frequency electrical current. Diathermy is used to seal the ends of blood vessels during surgery.

Discharge letter   A letter given to patients as they leave hospital which gives details of their treatment and any other information of which their family doctor should be aware.

Ectopic pregnancy   Development of a fetus which has implanted outside the uterus, usually in a fallopian tube. An ectopic pregnancy is dangerous for the woman concerned, and the fetus cannot develop normally.

Efferent duct   A duct which carries sperm from the seminiferous tubules in the testis to the epididymis.

Ejaculation   The sudden ejection of semen from the penis following sexual arousal.

Ejaculatory duct   The duct which carries sperm and semen from the seminal vesicles to the urethra in the penis.

Electrocardiogram (ECG)   A record of the activity of the heart as a series of electrical wave patterns produced as the muscles in the heart beat.

Electrocautery   The application of the electrically heated tip of an instrument to the ends of blood vessels to stop them bleeding. This process can also be used to remove the endometrium from the uterus in an attempt to treat some forms of menstrual problems.

Embolus (plural: **emboli**)   A blood clot, or an air bubble, which blocks a blood vessel.

Endometrium   The vascular layer lining the uterus, part of which is shed during menstruation.

Epididymis   A mass of tissue attached to the border of the testis which is composed of tightly coiled efferent ducts carrying sperm produced within the testis.

Epididymitis   Inflammation of the epididymis.

Epidural anaesthetic   A local anaesthetic which is injected into the space around the spinal cord and numbs the back, legs and lower abdomen.

Fallopian tube   The tube through which ova pass on their way from an ovary to the uterus.

Family planning clinic   A clinic staffed by doctors and nurses specially trained to give advice on birth control and related matters. The services of family planning clinics are provided free under the NHS.

Femidom   A type of condom for use by women which consists of a polyurethane sheath attached between two flexible rings. It can be inserted by a woman into her vagina before sexual intercourse to collect sperm and prevent them entering the uterus. The condom can only be used once.

Fertilisation   The union of an ovum and a sperm to form an embryo.

Fetus (also **Foetus**)   A developing embryo.

Fixed Price Care   A system used by some private hospitals in which a fixed price is given for a particular operation and for some specific hospitalisation costs it is likely to involve.

Follicle-stimulating hormone (FSH)   A hormone which stimulates the production of ovarian follicles. It is produced by the pituitary gland at the base of the brain.

Forceps   A pincer-like surgical instrument used for holding or compressing tissue or an object.

Fundus (of uterus)   The part of the body of the uterus above the connections of the fallopian tubes.

General anaesthetic   A drug which induces sleep so that there is no sensation in any part of the body.

Genitalia   The reproductive organs, particularly the external ones such as the penis and testes.

Granuloma   A swelling composed of granulation tissue.

Gynaecologist   A doctor who specialises in the diagnosis and treatment of diseases affecting women.

Haematoma   A blood-filled swelling. Haematomas can form after surgery if a blood vessel continues to bleed. When the blood is spread in the tissues it appears as a bruise.

HIV/Human immunodeficiency virus   A micro-organism associated with the development of the disease known as AIDS.

Hormone   A chemical substance produced in one part of the body which passes via the bloodstream to another part where it has its effect. Different hormones control different functions within the body.

Hysterectomy   The surgical removal of the uterus.

Implantation   The embedding of a fertilised ovum, normally into the wall of the uterus.

Incision   A cut or wound made by a sharp instrument, such as during an operation.

Induction agent   A drug which induces sleep.

Inguinal canal   The canal through which the testes normally pass before birth from their position near the kidneys to the scrotum.

Inhalational anaesthetic   A drug in the form of a gas which is breathed in through a face mask.

Intra-uterine contraceptive device (IUCD)   See **Coil**.

Intramuscular   Within a muscle. An intramuscular injection introduces a substance directly into a muscle.

Intravenous   Within a vein. An intravenous injection introduces a substance directly into a vein.

Introitus   The opening of the vagina in the vulva.

'Keyhole' surgery   A colloquial name for minimally invasive or laparoscopic surgery.

Laparoscope   A telescope-like instrument with a light source and camera attached which can be introduced into the abdominal cavity. It allows the surgeon to examine the internal organs without having to make a large incision. The inside of the body can be seen on a video screen within the operating theatre.

Laparoscopy   Surgery carried out with the aid of a laparoscope. It involves making a series of small incisions in the body wall through which the laparoscope and surgical instruments can be inserted.

Laparotomy   An operation in which a long incision is made in the abdomen so that the surgeon can see into the abdominal cavity.

Levonorgestrel   A synthetic hormone; a type of progestogen.

Ligament   A band of fibrous tissue connecting bones; also a strand of membrane which connects the abdominal organs to each other or to the abdominal wall. The **broad ligament** is attached to either side of the uterus and to the ovaries.

Lithotomy position   A position used for some gynaecological operations in which the woman lies on her back with her legs apart and her feet resting in stirrups.

Local anaesthetic   A drug which blocks the sensation in the area around which it is injected, causing numbness.

'Lurking sperm'   The term used for the very small number of sperm which may remain in the semen samples of a man who has undergone a vasectomy.

Luteinising hormone (LH)   The hormone produced by the pituitary gland in the brain and involved in the process of ovulation.

Maintenance agent   A drug which keeps you asleep.

Medical history   Details of someone's past health, including illnesses, operations, allergies etc.

Menopause   The time at which spontaneous menstruation ceases in women at the end of their natural reproductive life.

Menstrual cycle   The approximately monthly pattern of bleeding and the days between episodes of bleeding. Day 1 of the menstrual cycle is the day on which bleeding starts, and the last day is the day before the start of the next episode of bleeding. If heavy bleeding is preceded by very light bleeding or spotting, it is the first day of the heavy bleeding which is day 1 of the cycle.

Menstruation   The discharge of blood from the uterus which occurs at approximately monthly intervals in women throughout their reproductive life, but which ceases during pregnancy and lactation.

Minimally invasive surgery   Another name for laparoscopic surgery which involves a much less invasive technique than conventional surgery.

Monitoring device   Equipment used to watch over (monitor) the various activities of the body such as heart beat, breathing rate etc.

Myometrium   The muscle layer in the wall of the uterus.

Named nurse   A nurse allocated to a particular patient who is responsible for that patient's nursing care throughout their stay in hospital. The idea of 'named nurses' was introduced under the terms of the Government's Patients' Charter.

Natural family planning   There are various methods of natural family planning, which all involve refraining from sexual intercourse during the fertile phase of a woman's menstrual cycle, thus avoiding conception.

Nausea   A feeling of sickness.

'Nil by mouth'   A term used to mean that nothing – neither food nor drink – must be swallowed in the hours before an operation.

Non-absorbable suture/stitch   A stitch made of a material which will not dissolve. Non-absorbable sutures need to be removed once the wound has healed or, if they are used internally, remain in place forever.

Noristerat   A contraceptive injection, the effects of which last for about eight weeks.

Norplant   A newly available contraceptive in the form of an implant, about the same size as a matchstick. It can be inserted under the skin, usually in the arm, and releases progestogen into the body. It is effective for about five years and, when removed, fertility returns within a few days.

Obesity   An excessive amount of fat in the body. Obesity is a non-specific term which is being replaced by a figure calculated from height and weight measurements and known as **body mass index (BMI)**.

Oestrogen   A hormone which in women stimulates sexual development at puberty and changes in the endometrium during the menstrual cycle. It is produced by the ovaries and by the adrenal glands situated above the kidneys.

Oral contraception   A method of contraception which involves taking pills by mouth.

Ovarian cyst   A fluid-filled swelling which enlarges the ovary. Small ovarian cysts are normal and common. Larger ones can cause problems and may have to be removed surgically.

Ovarian follicle   A small cavity containing an ovum which is produced in an ovary.

Ovary   A female reproductive organ which produces ova and hormones.

Ovulation   The release of an ovum. Ovulation occurs 14 days before the start of the next period.

Ovum (plural: **ova**)   A female egg before it has been fertilised by a sperm.

Penis   The male sexual organ which becomes enlarged and erect as a result of sexual arousal, and through which semen is ejected. Urine also leaves the body via the penis.

Period   The days of the menstrual cycle on which bleeding occurs.

Pomeroy's operation   A surgical procedure which is commonly used for female sterilisation. It involves tying an absorbable suture around the base of a loop made in each fallopian tube, and then cutting away a section of the looped tube above it. The suture gradually dissolves, leaving the two ends of the tube separated and closed off.

Port   A narrow tube which is inserted through a small hole in the body wall, for example in the abdomen during a laparoscopic operation. A valve is attached to this tube so that gas and surgical instruments can be introduced into and removed from the body cavity without the loss of the gas used to inflate it.

Post-operative   After an operation.

Pre-medication (Pre-med.)   Any drug which is given before another, e.g. a drug given before an anaesthetic to reduce the patients' anxiety by making them relaxed and drowsy.

Pre-operative   Before an operation.

Progesterone   A steroid which stimulates changes in the female reproductive organs, preparing them for pregnancy. The main changes are an increase in the blood supply in the lining of the womb so that it can support a fetus. There may also be a slight increase in the size of the breasts.

Progestogen Any drug which mimics the action of proges-terone.

Prostate gland A gland which surrounds the neck of the bladder and urethra in men, and which secretes a fluid which forms part of the semen. The prostate gland often becomes enlarged in elderly men, causing constriction of the urethra and thus retention of urine.

Puberty The time at which the sex glands become active. In girls, menstruation begins, the uterus, ovaries and vagina enlarge, and the breasts and pubic hair start to develop. In boys, the penis and testes enlarge, and sperm production begins. Hair starts to develop on the face, body and pubic region, and the voice deepens.

Pulmonary embolism A clot of blood or an air bubble which forms within the blood vessels of the lungs.

Recovery room A ward near an operating theatre where patients are taken to recover from the anaesthetic after surgery. The recovery room is staffed by nurses who are specially trained in this type of care.

Reversal (of sterilisation) A major and technically difficult surgical procedure by which an attempt is made to rejoin the cut ends of the fallopian tubes or vasa deferentia. The operation is not always successful, and in some cases cannot even be attempted.

Salpingectomy The surgical removal of the fallopian tubes.

Scrotum The pouch of skin below the penis which contains the testes.

Segmental excision A surgical procedure involving the removal of a segment of each fallopian tube through an incision made in the abdomen. Pomeroy's operation is a common means of performing this process.

Semen A fluid containing sperm together with secretions from the prostate gland and seminal vesicles.

Seminal vesicle A coiled tube which stores semen.

Seminiferous tubule   A tube which is tightly coiled within the testis and in which sperm are produced. Each testis contains several hundred seminiferous tubules.

Side-effect   An unwanted effect which accompanies another disease or treatment.

Speculum   Any instrument used to inspect a passage or tube, commonly the vagina.

Sperm   The mature male cell containing male genetic material capable of developing into a new individual when united with a female egg. It consists of a small head region, a short middle piece, and a motile tail which enables the sperm to swim.

Spermatic cord   The cord in the scrotum which carries sperm from the testis, together with arteries and veins.

Spermicide   A substance which can kill sperm.

Sphincter   A ring-shaped muscle surrounding the opening to a tube which is able to open and close to control the entry of substances into it.

Spinal anaesthetic   A drug which is injected between the bones of the spine into the space around the nerves, and which causes numbness in the legs and lower abdomen.

Step-down ward   A ward to which day-case patients go in some hospitals to recover before going home after an operation.

Sterilisation   A procedure which makes someone unable to reproduce. Sterilisation is used as a form of contraception. It involves surgery to prevent the passage of ova or sperm, thus preventing fertilisation occurring.

Suppository   A cone-shaped medical preparation, made of wax or gelatine and containing a drug, which can be inserted into the body, usually the rectum. Although solid at room temperature, the suppository melts at the temperature of the body.

Surgery   The treatment of disease or injury by operation.

Suture   A surgical stitch or row of stitches. Sutures can be absorbable or non-absorbable, the latter normally having to be removed once the wound has healed.

Testis   The male reproductive organ in which sperm develop; the testicle.

Thrombosis   The coagulation of blood within a vein or artery to produce a blood clot.

Thrombus   A blood clot which forms in, and remains in, a blood vessel or the heart.

Trocar   A sharp instrument through which other instruments can be inserted into a body cavity.

Tubal ligation/occlusion   A surgical procedure involving the tying off of the fallopian tubes, usually using special rings or clips.

Undescended testicles   The failure of the testes to descend spontaneously before birth from their position near the kidneys, through the inguinal canal to the scrotum.

Urethra   The tube through which urine passes as it is discharged from the bladder.

Urine retention   The inability to empty the bladder, which can occur, for example, following an operation in the abdominal cavity.

Urological surgeon   A doctor who has specific training in, and experience of, problems of the urinary system.

Urology   The study of the urinary system.

Uterus   The muscular organ in which an embryo develops during pregnancy; the womb.

Vagina   The canal between the uterus and the vulva.

Vas deferens (plural: **vasa deferentia**)   The tube which carries sperm from the testis to the penis.

Vasectomy   The surgical removal of a section of the vasa deferentia which is performed to render a man sterile.

Vulva   The external female organs, including the openings of the vagina and urethra, the clitoris and the labia.

Womb   The uterus.

How to complain

If you are unhappy about anything that has occurred – or, indeed, that has not occurred – during your stay in hospital, there are several possible paths to follow if you want to make a complaint.

However, before you set the complaints machinery in motion, you should give careful thought to what is involved. Once a formal complaint has been made against a doctor and the complaints procedure has begun, there is little chance of stopping it.

If you think you have a genuine grievance, do try to talk to the person concerned, explaining as clearly and unemotionally as possible what it is that you feel has gone wrong. If you do not feel you want to discuss things directly, you can always present your case in a letter.

The vast majority of doctors – GPs and hospital doctors – are dedicated, conscientious and hard working. They really do have their patients' best interests at heart, and many work very long hours each week, night and day. The many hours of overtime worked by junior hospital doctors, for example, are compulsory and poorly paid.

A complaint against a doctor is usually a devastating blow, which can cause considerable stress. Of course, if something has gone wrong during your medical treatment, you may also have suffered stress and unhappiness, but before you make an official complaint, do consider whether your doctor's actions have really warranted what many would see as a 'kick in the teeth'.

The best approach is to make a polite and reasoned enquiry to the person concerned. However angry or irritated you may feel, you are likely to find that a complaint made aggressively – however justified this may seem – is unlikely to achieve much.

If you wish to bring something to the attention of hospital staff which does not seem serious enough to warrant a formal complaint, the 'suggestion boxes' now used by many hospitals may be a useful alternative.

Leaflets and other information giving details of all the appropriate councils and complaints procedures and how they work can be obtained from your hospital or local health authority. A Citizens' Advice Bureau or Community Health Council will also be able to give you information about what to do and who to go to for help if you have any problems with the offices mentioned here.

HOSPITAL STAFF

If your complaint concerns something that has happened during your stay in hospital, and for some reason you are unable to approach the person directly concerned, you can talk to the ward sister or charge nurse, the hospital doctor on your ward, or the senior manager for the department or ward. Many complaints can be dealt with directly by one of these people, but if this is not possible, they will be able to refer you to the appropriate authority.

THE HOSPITAL GENERAL MANAGER

If you are intimidated by the thought of speaking to one of the people mentioned above, you can write to the hospital's General Manager, sometimes called the Director of Operations or Chief Executive. The General Manager has responsibility for the way the hospital is run.

The Government's Patients' Charter states that anyone making a complaint about an NHS service must receive a 'full and prompt written reply from the Chief Executive or General Manager'. You should therefore receive an immediate response to your letter, and your complaint should be fully investigated by a senior manager.

The hospital switchboard, or any medical or clerical staff at the hospital, should be able to give you the General Manager's name and office address. If you would prefer to do so, you can make an appointment to speak to him or her rather than writing a letter.

Depending on how serious your complaint is, you should receive either a full report of the investigation into it, or regular letters telling you what is happening until such a report can be made.

Do make sure you keep copies of all letters you write and receive concerning your complaint.

DISTRICT HEALTH AUTHORITY

If the treatment you require is not available in your area, or the waiting list is very long, you can contact your local District Health Authority. The District Health Authority is able to deal with complaints concerning the provision of services, rather than with those resulting from something going wrong with your treatment. Arrangements can sometimes be made for you to have treatment elsewhere where waiting lists are shorter, if this is what you want.

Your NHS authority should produce a leaflet to explain how it deals with complaints. This will be available at your hospital or clinic. If you have any difficulty finding out who to contact, write to the General Manager of the hospital. Someone at the hospital will be able to tell you which health authority covers the area in which you live.

COMMUNITY HEALTH COUNCIL

If you feel that you would like independent advice and assistance, you can obtain this from your local Community Health Council. Someone from the Community Health Council will be able to explain the complaints procedures to you, help you to write letters to the hospital, and also come with you to any meetings arranged between hospital representatives and yourself. Again, the address of the Community Health Council for your area can be obtained from a hospital or local telephone directory.

REGIONAL MEDICAL OFFICER

If your complaint concerns the standard of *clinical* treatment you received in hospital, and the paths you have already taken have not led to a satisfactory conclusion, you can take it to the Regional Medical Officer for your area.

FAMILY HEALTH SERVICES AUTHORITY

Any complaint about a GP which you have been unable to sort out with the doctor in question can be reported to the Family Health Services Authority. Such complaints should be made within 13 weeks of the incident occurring. Again, your local Community Health Council will be able to give you advice, help you make your complaint, and help you to write letters etc.

HEALTH SERVICE COMMISSIONER

If all else has failed, you can take your complaint to the Health Service Commissioner, who deals with complaints made by individuals against the NHS. The Commissioner is independent of both the NHS and the Government, being responsible to Parliament.

The Health Service Commissioner is able to deal with complaints concerning the failure of an NHS authority to provide the service it should – a failure which has caused you actual hardship or injustice. However, you must have taken your complaint up with your local health authority first. If you have not received a satisfactory response within a reasonable time, you must enclose copies of *all* the relevant letters and documents as well as giving details of the incident itself when writing to the Health Service Commissioner. The Health Commissioner is not able to investigate complaints about clinical treatment.

You must also contact the Health Service Commissioner within *one* year of the incident occurring, unless there is some valid reason why you have been unable to do so.

There is a different Health Service Commissioner for each country within the United Kingdom.

Health Service Commissioner for England
Church House
Great Smith Street
London SW1P 3BW
Telephone: 0171 276 2035

Health Service Commissioner for Scotland
Second Floor
11 Melville Crescent
Edinburgh EH3 7LU
Telephone: 0131 225 7465

Health Service Commissioner for Wales
4th Floor
Pearl Assurance House
Greyfriars Road
Cardiff CF1 3AG
Telephone: 01222 394621

Office of the Northern Ireland Commissioner for Complaints
33 Wellington Place
Belfast BT1 6HN
Telephone: 01232 233821

TAKING LEGAL ACTION

The legal path is likely to be an expensive one, and should be a last resort rather than a starting point. In theory, everyone has a right to take legal action. However, unless you have very little money and are entitled to Legal Aid, or a great deal of money, you are unlikely to be able to afford this costly process. The outcome of legal action can never be assured, and the possible cost if you lose your case should be borne in mind.

If you do think you have grounds for compensation for injury caused as a result of negligence, advice can be sought from:

The Association for the Victims of Medical Accidents (AVMA)
1 London Road
Forest Hill
London SE23 3TP
Telephone: 0181 291 2793.

Someone from the AVMA will be able to give you free and confidential legal advice about whether you have a case worth pursuing. They will also be able to recommend solicitors with training in medical law who may be prepared to represent you.

SUMMARY

Do tell nursing or other medical staff if you are not happy about *any* aspect of your care in hospital. They may be able to deal with your problem immediately. But do remember, if your complaint is about a serious matter, or if you are not satisfied with the response you receive, you are entitled to pursue it through all the levels that exist to deal with such problems.

Index

abscess   78
anaesthetics
  allergy to   52
  general   51–6
    recovery from   74, 83
    risks of   56
    side-effects of   55–6, 83
  inhalational   52
  intravenous   52
  local   50–1
anaesthetist   41
  ward visit by   46, 51–2
anti-embolism
    stockings   47–8
Association for the Victims of
  Medical Accidents   127

bladder catheter   64, 77, 82
blood clots   47
bruising, after
  vasectomy   72–3, 79–80

carbon dioxide, for
    laparoscopy   65
  post-operative effects
    of   75
cervical smear test   30
chest infection   79
clips, fallopian   66, 67–8

coil (*see* contraceptives,
    IUCDS)
Community Health
    Council   125
complications, post-
    operative   78–9
  after tubal ligation   82–4
  after vasectomy   79–82
consent form   31–2, 46
contraception
  barrier methods   16–19
  calendar method   18
  cervical caps   16, 17
  cervical mucus method   18
  condoms   18–19
  diaphragms   16, 17
  double-check method   19
  implants   14–15
  injections   14
  IUCDS   15
  oral   13–14
  spermicides   19
  sponges   19
  temperature method   18
culdotomy   61

day-case surgery   37
deep vein thrombosis (*see*
    blood clots)

129

Depo-provera   14
diathermy   61
District Health
    Authority   124
doctors, hospital   40–1
    ward visits by   45–6
drugs   45
    allergies to   52

ectopic pregnancy   15, 25
efferent duct   8
ejaculation   9, 10
ejaculatory duct   9
electrocautery   44
emboli   47
epididymis   8

fallopian tubes   2
    closure of   10 (*see also* tubal
        ligation/occlusion)
Family Health Services
    Authority   125
Femidom   18
Fixed Price Care   86–8
follicle-stimulating
    hormone   6

haematoma   79, 80
Health Service
    Commissioner   125–7
hospital
    admission to   44–5
        private   89–90
    length of stay in   41–2
Hospital General
    Manager   123
hysterectomy   11, 26

incisions
    for tubal ligation   66, 69,
    for vasectomy   60
inguinal canal   7
inhalational anaesthetic   52
intravenous anaesthetic   52

laparoscope   62
laparoscopic
    sterilisation   62–8
    failure of   34, 67
    post-operative recovery
        from   75–6
laparotomy   68–71
    failure of   34
    post-operative recovery
        from   76–7
lurking sperm   35
luteinising hormone   6

menopause   6
menstruation   4–6, 11
    effects of sterilisation
        on   31
    problems of   26

natural family
    planning   19–20
'nil by mouth'   46–7, 53
Noristerat   14
Norplant   14–15
nurses   38–9
    in recovery room   55

obesity, risks of for general
    anaesthetic   48
ova   1

ovarian follicle   1
ovaries   1–2
ovulation   1
    after sterilisation   11
    role of in natural family
        planning   19–20

pain, post-operative
    after tubal ligation   75, 76,
        83
    after vasectomy   60, 72,
        82
    in shoulder   75
    relief of   56–7
penis   9
periods, *see* menstruation
physical examinations   27–30
    by student doctors   32
Pomeroy's operation   69
pregnancy   27
    after tubal ligation   25,
        84
    ectopic   15, 25
progesterone   2
    in oral
        contraceptives   13–14
prostate gland   6

recovery room   55
Regional Medical Officer   125
regret   23
    after vasectomy   82
    after tubal ligation   83
reversal of sterilisation   32–4
rings, fallopian   66, 67

salpingectomy   25

scrotum   7, 8
segmental excision   10–11,
        68–71
semen samples   25, 74
seminal vesicle   8–9
seminiferous tubules   8
sexual intercourse
    after vasectomy   73
    after laparoscopy   76
    after laparotomy   77
shaving, before
        vasectomy   47
shoulder pain, after
        laparoscopy   75
smoking, risks of for general
        anaesthesia   48
speculum, use of
    for cervical smear test   30
    for vaginal examination   29
sperm   8, 10
    production of after
        vasectomy   12
sperm antibodies   81
spermatic cord   7
sperm granuloma   81
step-down ward   55
stitches
    after vasectomy   73
    after laparoscopy   75
    after laparotomy   76
swelling (*see also* haematoma)
    after vasectomy   72–3, 79

testes   7–8
thrombo-embolic deterrent
        stockings   47–8
thrombosis, *see* blood clots

tubal
   ligation/occlusion   10–11,
      24–5, 61–71
   contraindications   23–4
   failure of   34
   general anaesthesia
      for   51–4
   local anaesthesia for   51
   post-operative recovery
      from   74–7
   reversal of   32–4

urethra, male   6
urine retention   77, 82
uterus   3–4

vagina   4
vaginal examination   29

vas deferens   8
vasectomy   11–12, 24–5,
      58–60
   contraindications   21–2,
      23–4
   failure of   35
   general anaesthesia
      for   51–4
   local anaesthesia for   50
   post-operative recovery
      from   72–4
   reversal of   32–3, 34

work, returning to
   after tubal ligation   75–6
   after vasectomy   73
wound infection   78
   after vasectomy   80